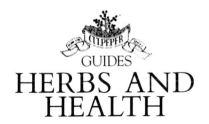

GUIDES
HERBS AND HEALTH

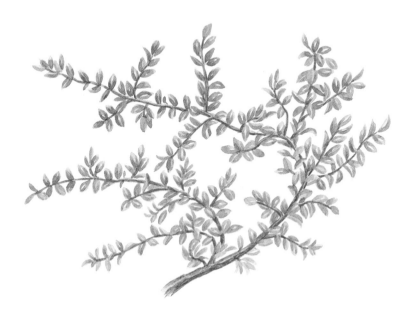

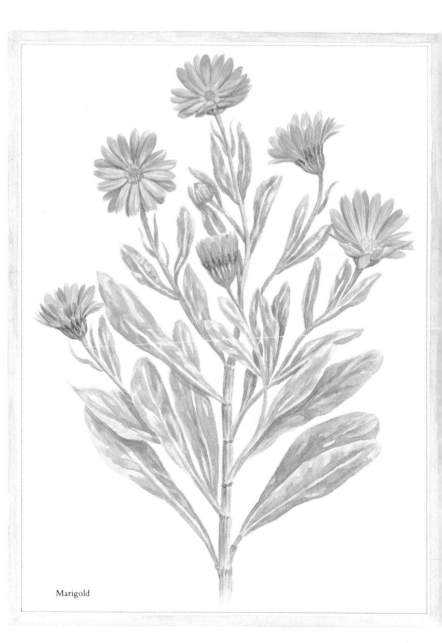

Marigold

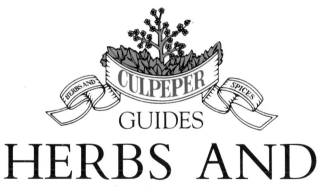

GUIDES

HERBS AND HEALTH

NICOLA PETERSON

Illustrated by
ROSAMUND GENDLE

General Editor
IAN THOMAS

SEAFARER

SEAFARER BOOKS
a division of Penguin Books USA Inc.
375 Hudson Street, New York, New York 10014

First American edition published in 1994 by Seafarer Books,
a division of Penguin Books USA Inc.

First Seafarer printing, April 1994

General Editor: Ian Thomas

Published in Great Britain in 1989 by Webb & Bower (Publishers)
Limited

Culpeper is a trademark of Culpeper Limited.

ISBN 0-8289-0857-5

Printed and bound in Great Britain by
BPC Hazell Books Ltd
A member of
The British Printing Company Ltd

10 9 8 7 6 5 4 3 2 1

Contents

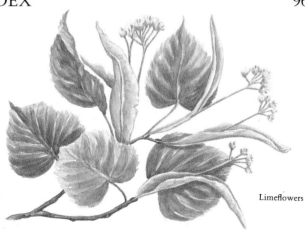

Limeflowers

FOREWORD

The increasing interest in herbal and other alternative medicine undoubtedly stems from people's experience of modern synthesized drugs: their effects upon themselves, their families and their friends. Millions of people take chemical tranquilizers every day. In the past, their parents coped. Simple aches and sprains are now relieved with cortisone. Hormone treatments are common.

Nicola Peterson writes simply and clearly about how you can use simple herbal treatments as home remedies. You may be surprised to find some of the herbs recommended are already in your kitchen. But this is not a homespun herbal. Nicola Peterson is a qualified medical herbalist with practical experience of what concerns her patients and how she can help.

There is a fundamental difference between modern synthesized drugs and modern herbalism. The modern pharmacist seeks to identify and isolate what he or she regards as the one "active" element in the plant or chemical substance. Once isolated, the effects of this concentrated ingredient can be tested, the final drug prescribed and produced in profitable quantities. The modern herbalist believes that it is the whole herb not just one ingredient in it which helps the disease in your body; that the other components of the plant buffer the more active ingredients. Herbal remedies are less concentrated. They are rightly regarded as safer, more gentle and less toxic.

This does not mean however that all herbs are totally harmless. If that were so, they would probably be ineffectual as medicines. Wherever in the book you see the word CAUTION, please read the notes carefully. A medicine is taken to correct an imbalance of the body's functions. No medicine, herbal or otherwise, should be necessary for too long. The herbal remedies in the book are for simple everyday conditions. Always consult your doctor or qualified herbal practitioner if you suspect any serious health disturbance or have any chronic warning symptoms.

Ian Thomas

INTRODUCTION

The folklore of herbal medicine, which our grandparents were familiar with through economic necessity (the doctor and his medicines being too costly for most people), has declined today, for the majority of people have access to low-cost medical treatment. Thus to someone not familiar with the profession, herbal medicine may seem to have connections with superstition and a non-scientific, "mystic" approach to medicine. Nothing could be further from the truth.

The current professional qualification for the National Institute of Medical Herbalists (England) is achieved after successfully completing a four-year training course. It includes the standard medical subjects of anatomy, physiology and diagnosis. Beyond this, there is also teaching on the philosophy behind the natural approach to health and illness, and extensive courses on the use of herbal remedies, including the subjects of pharmacy and pharmacology (the science of investigating the therapeutic benefits of plant constituents).

Specialist areas which may be particularly relevant to the herbal practitioner, such as dermatology and gynecology, are covered in depth. A long period of clinical training is required, to ensure that the student is highly competent in the use of standard diagnostic equipment and techniques. Examinations in this and the academic subjects must all be passed before membership in the Institute is granted. At this stage, the new practitioner, as in all types of medicine, has a basis on which to build a career – and a lot more to learn from experience!

The basic difference between the majority of orthodox doctors and the medical herbalist lies in the approach to health and illness. Most natural practitioners accept a "vitalistic" rather than a "mechanistic" principle – that is, all living organisms may be likened to complex machines to a certain degree, but one cannot stop there. Unlike machines all life has the potential for self-healing. There is also the "self-balancing" principle, known as "homeostasis," whereby living organisms readjust to changes that affect their functioning. This minimizes any long-term damage by maintaining a "steady-state" within the body. Herbal practitioners respect these wonderful natural abilities and use medicines to support rather than disrupt this natural process.

It follows that herbal practitioners see a state of health as a far more positive condition than a mere absence of disease – the physical, mental, and spiritual aspects of a person must be at their optimum to enable the full enjoyment of life. This is the core of the "holistic" ideal of medicine, an ideal which we, the herbal practitioners, strive to put into practice for the benefit of each of our patients.

It is often said that herbal practitioners treat the patient rather than the disease. This may be difficult to understand in a culture where "X" drug is given to treat "Y" illness. This may be very successful, rapidly so in certain cases, but it does not provide the answer for the patients who end up coming to see me. The extensive notes I make about all aspects of a patient's health, which I have heard discussed as mere "clerking" by some doctors, is really essential to the type of diagnosis I am seeking. This is quite different from the orthodox diagnostic approach of identifying a disease or syndrome, and then looking for the drug with which to treat it. What I am looking for is, for example, how far a person's nervous system is contributing to their symptoms or their circulation, or their kidney and bowel function, and so on, through all the systems of the body, to assess their involvement in the apparent problem.

This approach is based on sound physiological principles: it recognizes the interdependence of all functions of the body, and accepts that if one system is not working properly it will have consequences for the others. For instance, the kidneys deal with the removal of toxic waste from the body: if they are not working efficiently, the result can be skin inflammation or arthritic disorder, due to irritants accumulating in the body rather than being expelled in the normal way.

The prescriptions I make for my patients may contain up to eight different liquid herbal extracts to help restore the balance to the different body systems which have been found to be unhealthy. The ease with which remedies can be combined is one of the great strengths of herbal medicine: it effects an improvement which the patient often describes as "feeling better in myself even before the specific symptoms may have cleared." It is the skill of creating the best combinations for each individual patient's needs that is the essential art of the professional herbalist. In this book my aim is to convey a much simplified form of this approach, which can then be understood and put into practice by the lay person. My approach is faithful to the principles of the holistic method, and by being so it stands a better chance of success than the use of isolated herbal remedies. But the methods described here are limited in breadth and depth compared with the treatment that a professional herbalist would give to a patient.

Another aspect of the holistic view of maintaining good health is concerned with what people can do for themselves, with correct diet and exercise, before ever considering medical therapy. Again, this is connected with a positive view of health which emphasizes the importance of giving the body what it needs to keep in good shape.

For most people, a fairly plain whole-food diet is to be recommended. A wide range of fruit and vegetables should be eaten regularly – these contain a large amount of water and fiber and as a result are non-concentrated in the nutritional value they supply. The fiber is valuable in itself because it is *not* absorbed – it adds bulk to the food passing through the digestive tract, thus giving the muscles that push the food along an easier job. This type of diet may need to be revised for people who have very sensitive digestive systems; excess fiber can be too irritating for some people and certain fruits can cause indigestion. Suspected fruit and vegetables should be avoided and replaced by those that are more easily tolerated.

Cereals, beans and nuts represent a more concentrated source of nutrition than fruit and vegetables. Most people can take them freely, although again the fiber content in whole-grain cereals can be an irritant. I am not in favor of taking extra bran in the diet – this is actually a "refined" product, as it is one isolated part of the grain, without the balance of the whole. If possible, the whole-grain forms of flour, pasta and rice should be used, as they contain much more nourishment (and taste!) than the white equivalent.

Animal foods – including milk and its products, eggs, meat and fish – are the most concentrated foods available and are best eaten only in relatively small amounts for a well-balanced diet. They all have the same benefits: high-quality proteins, plenty of vitamins, minerals and energy value. But animal foods also contain large amounts of undesirable saturated fats. Human beings are not adapted for dealing with large amounts of fats – they block the blood vessels, causing problems such as angina, and the inherent energy that is not used is deposited as fat in our bodies.

The other personal responsibility we have – exercise – is now becoming recognized as essential to the well-being of us all, not just the prerogative of the "sporty" few. Our bodies are designed to be on the move most of the time, and generally work best under such conditions. Exercise stimulates the circulation, the lungs, the digestion, various eliminative processes and burns up calories that would otherwise be stored as fat. The average person needs to walk about six miles a day to preserve optimum health; but this can be condensed into half an hour's steady, non-stop exercise on alternate days. Swimming, cycling, jogging or even a really brisk walk will fulfill the requirements by providing a stimulus to which the body will respond.

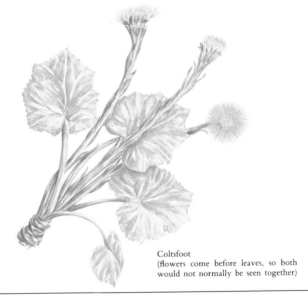

Coltsfoot
(flowers come before leaves, so both would not normally be seen together)

QUESTIONS AND ANSWERS

Now that the general principles of holistic medicine have been covered, I would like to discuss herbal medicine in particular. It differs from orthodox medicine in several important practical ways, and I think the best way of explaining these differences is in the form of answers to questions I am frequently asked. I do recommend that you read this part of the book before turning to the reference section: it will help you to understand more fully how and why herbs can be used as medicines.

QUESTIONS I AM FREQUENTLY ASKED
Isn't herbal medicine very old-fashioned?

Herbal medicine is one of the oldest skills still practiced: just about every human culture in history has had some version of it. Of course, before the modern developments in science were made, herbalists did not know why their plant remedies worked, and they may have made guesses at explanations which now seem quaintly inaccurate (as were many of the "orthodox" medical theories in the past!). This was less important, though, than the demonstration that the remedies *did* work – and this part of the knowledge is what has been passed down to present-day practitioners. Contemporary herbalists, as well as doctors, have benefited from medical science: we understand more about how the body works in health, what happens when it is diseased, and how and why the herbal remedies help to correct the processes that have gone wrong. Many plants have been analyzed to reveal their most important therapeutic ingredients. All this relatively new knowledge has been added to the traditional knowledge of herbal medicine to produce better-informed practitioners who are able to benefit from the wealth of experience of previous generations. The plants still work in the same way that they have for thousands of years and practitioners still have the same respect for the wonderful natural healing powers of the body. In addition, a wealth of scientific knowledge about how the remedies work has greatly enriched the body of knowledge concerned with herbal medicine in the twentieth century.

Aren't herbs really just like weak drugs?

Many of the drugs used in the twentieth century were originally discovered in plant material. The drugs have been isolated and extracted from the plants and given as single substances for their therapeutic actions. The advantage of this is that dosages can be measured very accurately, and the results of clinical trials of the drug can be easily interpreted. The great disadvantage, in the herbalists' opinion, is that all the other valuable therapeutic properties of the plant are ignored. Often there may be several similar substances in one plant which all contribute to the characteristic action. There may be widely differing constituents, with individually different actions, that help give the plant a number of therapeutic uses. Some constituents may have a modifying effect on each other; for instance, one might activate another to give the therapeutic benefit, as in **Garlic**, where an enzyme, released when the clove is crushed, helps to produce the active antiseptic principle. In **Meadowsweet**, the possible stomach irritation caused by its aspirin-like constituents is completely counteracted by others which actually make it beneficial for stomach disturbances.

Although the amount of each ingredient in a herbal remedy may vary from sample to sample, it is the overall balance of different constituents that is the most beneficial aspect of using plants as medicine. They may not work as quickly as orthodox single-substance drugs, but they are very well tolerated by the body and work at the body's own natural pace of change, often using reflexes already existing within the normal pattern of body function to correct abnormalities and promote a state of true health.

Does herbal medicine have side effects?

This question has taken on a sinister importance in the last twenty-five years, since a number of orthodox drugs, at first thought to be near-miraculous, have been shown to cause many side effects. The term "iatrogenic illness" describes illnesses that are actually caused by the process of medical examination or treatment. The effects may range from minor discomfort to very serious problems; many sufferers may initially turn to herbal medicine to find relief from the effects of prescribed drugs.

It is very unlikely that anything like these side effects will occur with herbal medicine. The remedies included in this book have at least as much similarity with the plants we know as foods as with drugs: in fact, the two best-known herbal preparations, tea and coffee, are definitely thought to be at the more potent end of the range of plant remedies! Our bodies are well adapted to "processing" plant material – we eat it every day. What is beneficial to the body is absorbed and used and what is not needed is eliminated. Of course there are poisonous plants, but these are well documented – in folklore as well as in contemporary science – and avoided accordingly. Plants which may cause side effects if taken in excess are available only to qualified herbal practitioners and are not included in this book.

There may be the occasional case of an allergic reaction, in the same way that some people are allergic to certain foods. The reaction will only be transient, but if it occurs it may be necessary to change the remedies for ones which are more easily tolerated by the body.

Will herbal medicine have a bad reaction with ordinary drugs?

One of the strengths of herbal medicine is that it has a role to play in the treatment of many illnesses where orthodox drugs are alleviating only part of a particular problem. This is because most herbal remedies work in a completely different way from drugs: rather than being a single chemical that has one specific effect on a biochemical process, herbs have a more general effect which may nourish, relax, or stimulate a particular issue of the body. This helps to achieve a "normalizing" of the function of the tissue so that it can once again respond to the varying requirements of the body.

A few herbs work because of one or two very potent constituents, and the practitioner will be careful not to prescribe these if they are being given in isolated form as an orthodox treatment. For instance, the **Purple Foxglove** contains several heart stimulants; the main one used in orthodox medicine is digoxin – the dose of which is very critical. Potent herbal medicines of this nature are not included in this book.

Many patients turn to herbal medicine because they want to stop taking their prescribed drugs. My approach to achieving this aim is to prescribe herbal medicine to be taken alongside the drugs, until the symptoms have cleared. If the patient is then confident to try, preferably with the doctor's consent, a small reduction in the amount of drugs taken, he or she will have taken the first step towards eventually stopping the drugs altogether. It may, however, be a very slow process with serious and complex problems such as high blood pressure or arthritis.

A completely different situation is when someone may be quite happy with their orthodox treatment, but may be experiencing problems with minor illnesses, such as colds and coughs, during the course of it. In this instance, herbal remedies can be taken with complete confidence to treat these minor problems.

Can any illness be treated with herbal medicine?

Of course herbal remedies have their limitations – no one system of medicine is one hundred percent successful against all illnesses. My personal opinion is that herbal medicine, because of its flexibility and the breadth of its range of actions, is one of the most universally applicable systems we have. Problems may be minor or severe, straightforward or complex. Depending on what is occurring in the affected tissues, there will always be some way in which herbal medicines can help. The role of herbal medicine may be indirect, such as aiding the digestion, encouraging relaxation, or improving the circulation or eliminative functions. But deficiencies in any of these systems will be adding to the burden of disease the body is having to cope with. If these supplementary problems can be improved, the chances of recovery from the specific illness are significantly improved.

Can herbal medicine be used during pregnancy?

Medical practitioners generally agree that few, if any, medicines should be taken during pregnancy. Even though herbal remedies are very mild in their action, I also prefer to advise caution in their use. Do not try self-treatment – consult a professional if there is a real need. The professional herbalist will avoid those remedies which are likely to cause problems (however minor).

Some remedies in this book carry a note which advises specifically against use during pregnancy. I personally cannot recall any cases where actual harm has been done, but, as many herbs contain muscle-stimulating properties they are best avoided, as contractions in the uterine muscle are most undesirable until the last month of pregnancy. (With this in mind, also beware of laxatives of any kind.)

Many women experience trouble-free pregnancies and have no need of either orthodox or herbal medicine. Labor is, of course, a natural function of birth rather than an illness. However, there are certain remedies which can be taken for approximately four weeks before the baby is due, to ensure that the pelvic organs are in optimum condition to cope with the rigors of birth. **Raspberry leaves, Motherwort, Black Haw** and **Ginger** have been used for this purpose for generations. There is no objective measure against which success can be judged, as every labor differs in its intensity. All four remedies, however, are known to be beneficial in related gynecological problems, such as excessively painful menstruation, where the functional problem behind the pain is very similar.

Can fresh herbs be used, or must I get the dried form?
Always use fresh herbs where possible. They will have the greatest potency as none of the valuable essential oils will have evaporated – a common problem in a poorly dried sample. Well-known garden herbs such as **Thyme, Peppermint, Rosemary** and **Red Sage** are typical of those that can be used fresh. Many more can be grown – fresh **Comfrey**, for instance, is invaluable.

When using fresh material, it is important to know the correct time of year to gather it, as the constituents in each part of the plant will vary with the seasons. Generally, leaves are used or harvested when the plant is just starting to show its flower buds; flowers are used when they have formed, but before they have opened; and roots are taken up when the leaves and stems have died down in the late autumn.

Growing your own herbs is an especially rewarding aspect of gardening: they will make a beautiful garden, enrich your cooking, and provide for the needs of your health! In my opinion, growing your own plants is infinitely preferable to collecting them from the wild. We have limited wild areas and many rare species are now legally protected. Even if a plant is abundant, its situation may render it unsuitable for use – plants that grow by the roadside will be too polluted with car-exhaust fumes. There is also the problem of identification – occasionally, dangerous mistakes are made when a poisonous plant is mistaken for a medicinal variety.

Plants that are not indigenous will have to be imported and are therefore always used in the dried form. Drying, as well as reducing the bulk and weight of the plant, preserves its properties against breakdown by bacteria or molds, and is the traditional way of preparing plants that have to be transported over long distances.

The potency of a dried herb can be judged by its appearance and scent: leaves should be fairly green and if the plant is scented, the odor should still be detectable. If, for instance, a sample of **Peppermint** has lost the familiar scent, the valuable oil has been lost due to evaporation.

How long does a course of herbal medicine last?

The only way to answer this question is with another question: How long does an illness last? We can estimate the duration of treatment for self-limiting conditions such as colds and sore throats quite accurately. With more serious or complex problems, such as chest infections or sinusitis, it is not so easy. With long-term diseases like arthritis or eczema, the duration of the treatment will probably be months rather than weeks. In very few cases, so much damage may have been done already that complete health will never be restored. Herbal remedies, therefore, may be needed permanently to relieve rather than cure an illness.

In orthodox medicine it is not unusual to assume that people suffering from chronic (long-term) illnesses, such as high blood pressure or arthritis, will need treatment for the rest of their lives.

Herbal medicine is also well suited for long-term treatment, because of its low-impact nature on the body and the very low risk of side effects, even when it is prescribed for long periods of time. Having said that, however, I am often delighted at how quickly some apparently intractable problems respond to herbal treatment. My approach – and I would recommend this for self-treatment – when dealing with self-limiting conditions such as colds, coughs and sore throats, is to maintain the recommended dose of remedies until at least three days have passed since the symptoms have cleared.

The treatment of long-term illnesses is not so clear-cut. I would say maintain the recommended dose until the improvement, which may continue for several months initially, has reached a plateau and remained stable for about two months. If no further improvement is seen during this time (and in the absence of any relapse) the amount of medicine can be reduced to two-thirds of the previous dose. In practice, I usually recommend that the middle dose of medicine is omitted. This dosage should be maintained for another month. If the illness flares up again during this time, go back to three doses a day. If there are no problems, reduce the dose the following month to once a day; after another month, if all is still well, try without the medicine altogether. As I have stressed before, herbal remedies provide a flexible treatment – the medicine can always be adapted to your particular needs.

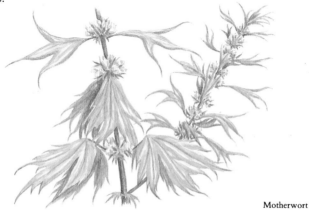

Motherwort

HOW TO USE THE
REFERENCE SECTIONS

This book is not intended to be either scholarly in its approach or comprehensive in the range of remedies included. Too much information can be as confusing and unhelpful for the novice as too little. In working out the amount of information to be included, I decided to list only the herbs that were generally well known and widely available. One or two more unusual varieties have been included, however, because of their outstandingly beneficial properties.

Rather than list the multitude of remedies that can be used in the treatment of a particular illness, I have mentioned at most only five, together with the reasons why they are so valuable to the holistic approach to the treatment of illness. My principal intention is to give clear information on a limited number of herbs so that the lay reader does not have to make decisions between numerous remedies of which he or she has no personal experience.

Of the illnesses mentioned, they are generally those that can be treated without professional advice – whether from a doctor or a herbalist. Individual cases will vary in terms of the severity of the problem – readers must use their own judgment. I must stress that anyone who is unsure of the nature of a particular problem should seek professional help rather than tackle it alone.

If you wish to treat an illness, look for the reference in the **"Everyday Illnesses"** section of the book. Note which remedies are recommended and then turn to the **"Alphabetical Herbal"** section to ascertain the method of preparation for use and the correct dosage.

How To Make The Herbal Preparations

Herbal remedies are far more flexible than conventional drugs. We know, for example, that to be effective, a specified amount of antibiotics must be taken for a specified number of days. In contrast, the dosage range of herbal treatment is very wide. Each individual may have different requirements, and different tolerances when it comes to taste! The following information provides the necessary guidelines for your first attempts at preparing herbal remedies.

INFUSION

Infusion is also known as tisane or tea. Traditionally, 25g (1oz) of the dried herb is placed in a crock pot, and 600ml (1pt) of boiling water is poured over it. The vessel is covered, and after about 10 minutes, the liquid is strained off and about $^1/_3$ of it taken, the rest being put aside for 2 further doses later in the day. In practice, this results in a very strong-tasting liquid. If the taste makes it impossible to drink, try a more dilute infusion of about 1 heaped teaspoon to 200ml ($^1/_3$pt) of water – enough for 1 dose. Make the infusion in the same way, then try adding honey or fruit juice. In some cases, such as when celery seeds are used, a savory flavoring, like yeast extract, is appropriate. Although this preparation will not be as strong, if it is taken regularly it will have the same benefit. There is no value in drinking a preparation that is so strong that a second dose cannot be tolerated.

Where a "weak infusion" is suggested, use about $^1/_2$ teaspoon of the herb to 200ml ($^1/_3$pt) of water; for a "strong infusion" use 2 teaspoons to 200ml ($^1/_3$pt) of water.

Infusions can be made from all soft plant material – leaves, flowers and berries.

DECOCTION

Decoction is the term given to heating a substance in water in order to extract the essence. In this preparation used for roots and barks, the traditional strength is 25g (1oz) of herb to 900ml (1¹/₂pt) of water. These are placed in a pan, brought to simmering point and left simmering for about 15 minutes, or until the amount of liquid has reduced to about 600ml (1pt) – giving the same final strength as the infusion. The extra time and heat softens up the woody material to enable the therapeutic ingredients to be drawn out into the liquid. As with the infusion, dilute if necessary and flavor to suit individual taste.

Preparing remedies for children

Young children should be given a quarter of the adult dose, and children between the ages of five and eleven should be given half the adult dose. It may be necessary to flavor with fruit juice to disguise the taste of the herb.

LOTIONS

Lotions may be made from either infusions or decoctions, depending on the plant material. It is important that the lotion should be well strained, particularly if it is to be used on the ears and eyes. A paper coffee filter will catch any tiny particles that are left in the lotion.

STEAM INHALATION

Add about 300ml (¹/₂pt) of strong infusion to 600ml (1pt) of recently boiled water; cover with a towel. Place the patient's head under the towel to inhale the steam through the nose and mouth. This is an excellent way of treating nasal and chest infections, as the volatile constituents of the remedies are delivered immediately to the relevant areas. The warm steam helps to loosen phlegm and catarrh, and has a soothing effect on inflamed respiratory membranes.

POULTICES

Poultices are made for application over the affected area, such as arthritic joints, inflamed muscles, bruises, etc. They are made by adding hot water to the herb to make a paste, and if necessary using a "binder" such as slippery elm powder or linseed meal.

When the right consistency is reached, spread the paste over a piece of flannel; apply to the skin and cover with wool, or similar material, to maintain the heat. The poultice can be kept in place until it starts to dry out or has lost all its heat.

The benefit of poulticing is twofold: the therapeutic benefit of the herb and the fact that the warmth and moisture help to soften the skin, thus allowing the plant constituents to be absorbed more easily. The heat also helps to relax the local muscles, easing tension and pain.

CAUTION: **Poultices should not be used on broken skin, as the warm moist conditions will enable any bacteria present to flourish. Poultices can be used on boils and abscesses to draw the infection to a focus, thus speeding up the process of discharge and resolution.**

GLOSSARY OF TERMS

THE MEDICINAL CONSTITUENTS OF PLANTS
Volatile Oils
The oil from each aromatic plant is formed from a number of volatile constituents, and the variation of these gives each plant its own characteristic scent. It may occur in leaves, flowers and seeds. Certain properties are common to all volatile oils: they are all antiseptic; they soothe the digestion and help prevent flatulence and griping; and many calm the nervous system.

Tannins
These help to harden soluble proteins, forming a protective surface over inflamed tissues. Internally, they calm over–activity in the digestive system, **but** they may also reduce absorption of protein if taken for too long. Externally, they will help staunch the flow of blood and reduce inflammatory swellings.

Sugars
These occur in plants as an energy source, along with starches. They form a part of the molecular structure of **glycosides**, which occur widely and have a range of individual therapeutic actions.

Mucilages

These are basically forms of cellulose which form a "slippery" or gel consistency when they absorb water. This has a soothing effect by mimicking the body's own protective mechanism of mucus production.

Bitters

These substances stimulate the taste buds, which in turn stimulate the appetite and digestive system via the vagus nerve. They also stimulate the liver in detoxifying treatments.

Alkaloids

These are plant constituents containing nitrogen – originally called "vegetable alkalis". They have wide-ranging effects on body functions, including the circulatory, nervous, digestive and respiratory systems. The best-known alkaloid is probably caffeine.

Resins

These are insoluble in water and therefore usually extracted in high-alcohol tinctures. They are antiseptic and antifungal.

Saponins

These produce a soapy consistency when added to water – **Soapwort** herb, for example, can be used as a mild soap. Some may cause some irritation to the stomach that produces a reflex loosening of phlegm in the lungs. Others have molecules similar to the natural steroid hormones of the body. These have anti-inflammatory actions and a tonic influence on the reproductive system – mainly in the female, though there are one or two traditionally used for the male.

Flavonoids

Flavenoids have a range of actions. Some complement Vitamin C function, and will help to strengthen the blood vessels; some help reduce muscle-spasm. They are frequently occurring plant constituents.

THE MEDICINAL ACTIONS OF PLANTS
Alterative

Traditionally known as "blood-purifiers", this range of remedies helps to improve the efficiency of the body's powers of elimination. Some work on the liver, some on the kidneys, some on the lymphatic system. This approach will help in any treatment where a "cleansing" action is needed; for instance if it is thought that toxic waste products, or ingested pollutants, have been accumulating in the body.

Anodyne

Anodyne remedies have a pain-reducing effect. Herbal remedies generally do not have a strong pain-killing action – the aim of the treatment is to achieve a positive state of health rather than simply dull the pain. There are one or two remedies, however, which have a gentle pain-relieving action, perhaps because of their relaxing effect on the nervous system.

Antispasmodic

This treatment helps to relieve the intensity of excessive muscular contraction. The basic function of muscle tissue is to contract to produce movement – this produces locomotion in the muscles attached to the skeleton. In the digestive tract it produces the contractions necessary to push the food through the "tubing" in the abdomen. If the muscles are overstimulated by the nerves controling them, or if there is any source of irritation to them, they may go into excessive contraction – spasms – known as cramp, or colic in the digestive system. Remedies having a muscle-relaxant effect are necessary to counteract this.

Aromatic

Aromatic plants have a notable scent, produced by the volatile oil in the plant. Due to the variety of constituents in the oil, no two plants will have the same scent, or exact therapeutic actions.

Astringent

The term astringent refers to a plant that has a tightening, anti-inflammatory action on tissues. Most astringent plants have this action due to the tannins they contain.

Expectorant

An expectorant will help the production and elimination of

phlegm from the lungs. There are two types: the irritant expectorants, of which **Ipecacuanha** is the best-known example; and the soothing expectorants such as **Coltsfoot**. The irritants work by reflex action from the stomach to the lungs; when the stomach lining is irritated, a reflex response is produced in the lungs – more mucus is produced as a protective mechanism. This is then cleared from the lungs by coughing – a means of getting rid of any harmful substances. The irritant properties of **Ipecacuanha** on the stomach are well known – in large doses it causes vomiting! The soothing expectorants have an apparently paradoxical action: soothing any irritations and inflammation in the lungs, but helping to loosen tight phlegm at the same time.

Laxative
Laxatives promote activity in the bowel. Many laxatives work on a reflex in the digestive tract: when the lining of the upper intestine (the duodenum) is irritated, the muscles in the bowel are stimulated by a nerve reflex to increase their activity. These laxatives work on the principle that the body is trying to speed up the elimination of the irritating substance to protect itself from further harm. The second type of laxative is one which works by creating more bulk of food for the muscles of the digestive tract to work on. The remedies in this group usually have a high starch or cellulose content, which when moistened swells to become a soft, slippery gel consistency. The lubricating action is another benefit, as it enables food to pass more easily along the digestive tract.

Tonic
Tonics have a strengthening, vitalizing effect on the target tissues. They work partly by nourishing, partly by stimulating existing reflex patterns of activity, to enable the affected tissues to cope more successfully with any demands or stress to which they may be subjected. Tonics help to support and restore normal body function.

ALPHABETICAL HERBAL

Common name: AGRIMONY
Botanical name: AGRIMONIA EUPATORIA
Family: ROSACEAE
Part used: Leaves and stems
Constituents and uses: Agrimony is a useful remedy for many digestive problems such as indigestion, overactive irritable bowel and diarrhea. It contains a soothing volatile oil, bitter substance to stimulate the appetite and digestive functions (useful in sluggish stomach and liver conditions) and tannins which have an astringent action. This gives an overall anti-inflammatory and anti-diarrheal action to the plant, which should therefore **not** be used in cases of constipation.

It can be taken as an infusion, 3 times a day.

Common name: ANGELICA
Botanical name: ANGELICA ARCHANGELICA
Family: UMBELLIFERAE
Part used: Leaf and root
Constituents and uses: This plant has a gentle warming stimulating action on the digestion, the lungs and the circulation. It can be safely used where stronger stimulants, such as **Ginger** or **Cayenne**, may be too irritating. The soothing and carminative volatile oil, giving the root in particular its characteristic scent, helps support the digestion and appetite. Bitters and astringents also contribute to this. **Angelica** helps to loosen phlegm in the lungs, and helps protect against the harmful influence of cold and damp in lung disease. As a general warming circulatory remedy, it may help in many conditions where poor circulation is a factor.

The leaves can be prepared as an infusion and the root as a decoction. It should be taken 3 times daily.

Common name: ANISEED
Botanical name: PIMPINELLA ANISUM
Family: UMBELLIFERAE
Part used: Dried fruit
Constituents and uses: **Aniseed** is well known for its sweet,

aromatic taste and scent. The volatile oil responsible for this has properties which soothe the digestion and will ease colic-type pains and flatulence. It will also help to reduce congestion and irritation in the lungs, by loosening tight phlegm and easing persistent dry coughs. It has an antiseptic action, useful in chest and digestive infections. The seeds may be crushed before infusing to make a pleasant and effective tea. Taken either before or after meals, it will reduce flatulence. A drop of the essential oil on a sugar cube or in a teaspoon of honey-water will have a similar effect.

Common name: ARNICA
Botanical name: ARNICA MONTANA
Family: COMPOSITAE
Part used: Flowers
Constituents and uses: This plant is for **external use only on unbroken skin**, due to its toxicity when taken internally. It is a most useful plant for dispersing bruises and swellings due to minor injuries when applied over the affected area, **provided that the skin is not broken**. The bruise will fade and the swelling subside much more rapidly than otherwise, giving quicker relief of pain and discomfort, and speeding the healing process. The plant contains essential oils, bitters and astringents. It is available in cream form which makes a very convenient application. The cream can be used after applying distilled **Witch Hazel** – which has a strong astringent anti-inflammatory action. Follow up by using **Comfrey** poultice or ointment to heal the injury as quickly as possible. An infusion can be made from the dried flowers and applied in the same way as the cream.

Common name: AVENS
Alternative common name(s): HERB BENNET
Botanical name: GEUM URBANUM
Family: ROSACEAE
Part used: Leaves and stems
Constituents and uses: One of the most useful astringent remedies to help settle over-activity in the bowel. It contains tannins, bitters and essential oils which all contribute to this action. It works directly on the digestive tract walls to reduce the irritation (which may be due to a variety of causes, such as infection, excessively

Angelica

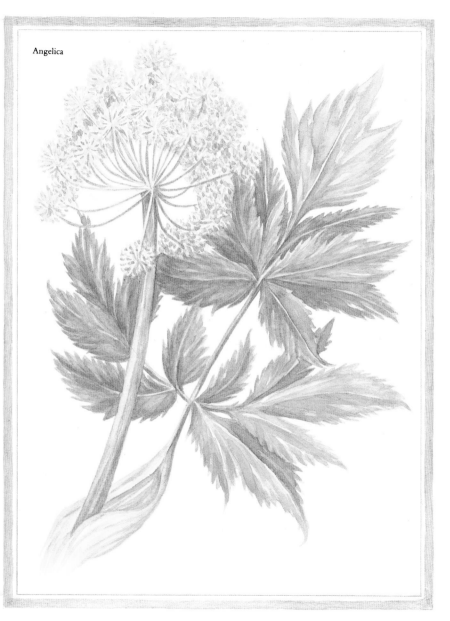

Aniseed

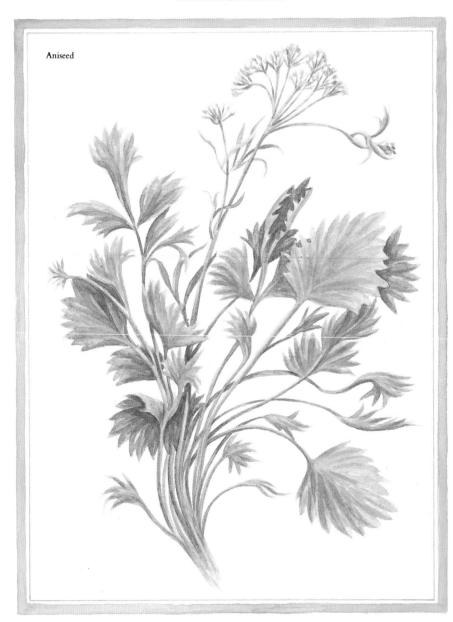

rich food, nervous tension, etc.) and thus soothes the muscular over-activity resulting from the irritation, which causes the hurrying of poorly digested food through to the bowel. It is effective in practically all "domestic" cases of diarrhea. In acute cases, an infusion should be taken every 3 hours for rapid benefits. It should be stopped as soon as the bowel activity is normal, as the strongly astringent action then becomes undesirable.

Common name: BALM OF GILEAD
Alternative common names(s): POPLAR BUDS
Botanical name: POPULUS GILEADENSIS
Family: SALICACEAE
Part used: Leaf buds harvested while tightly closed
Constituents and uses: The resin coating of these fragrant, sticky buds has a strong antiseptic and expectorant action. This remedy helps in all chest infections, to combat the infection directly and to help loosen the infected phlegm. The preparation of the buds is important – the resin does not dissolve well in water, so an infusion will not give the greatest benefit: an alcohol-based solution, such as made by adding 90ml vodka to 10ml water, is much more effective. Soak 20g (3/4oz) of the buds in this for 2 weeks, then strain and keep the liquid, which is a "tincture". This can then be taken internally in doses of up to 1 teaspoon, 3 times a day. Alternatively, 2 teaspoons of the tincture can be added to a bowl of boiling water, and the vapors inhaled to bring the evaporated constituents of the buds directly in contact with the lung tissue.
CAUTION: **The alcohol in this preparation makes it unsuitable for internal use for children.**

Common name: BEARBERRY
Botanical name: ARCTOSTAPHYLLOS UVA-URSI
Family: ERICACEAE
Part used: Leaves
Constituents and uses: This plant contains sugar-like substances called glycosides, the most significant being one called arbutin. When this enters the kidney, it is converted to an antiseptic substance which then helps destroy any harmful bacteria that may be causing a urinary infection. It is therefore specific for urinary

infections only, and does not damage the beneficial bacteria in the digestive system, as many orthodox antibiotic drugs do. It also avoids the "cystitis/antibiotics/thrush" cycle that troubles so many women.

Take the plant as an infusion 3 times daily, combined with diuretics to "flush through" the urinary system with extra fluid.

Common name: BETONY
Alternative common names(s): WOOD BETONY
Botanical name: BETONICA OFFICINALIS OR STACHYS BETONICA
Family: LABIATAE
Part used: Leaves and stems
Constituents and uses: **Betony** has a range of constituents which have a tonic effect on the nervous systems: it feeds and strengthens the nerves and contributes to a better tolerance of stress. It is particularly useful for headaches associated with nervous tension, and in conditions where long-term stress has caused general debility. Its bitter constituent makes it useful as a digestive tonic. Take as an infusion, 3 times a day.

Common name: BLACK HAW
Botanical name: VIBURNUM PRUNIFOLIUM
Family: CAPRIFOLIACEAE
Part used: Root bark
Constituents and uses: This plant is closely related to *Viburnum opulus*, the guelder rose which is also known as "cramp bark". Both have the ability to relax muscle spasms, but **Black Haw** is the chosen remedy for the excessive uterine muscle spasms that cause cramping pain during menstruation. It may reduced excessive blood loss, as it has astringent properties, and is helpful during menopause when blood loss may become very heavy and irregular.

A decoction should be taken 3 times daily, and the remedy may be combined with uterine tonics, circulatory remedies, or other uterine astringents as symptoms require.

Common name: BLADDERWRACK
Alternative common names(s): KELP
Botanical name: FUCUS VESICULOSUS

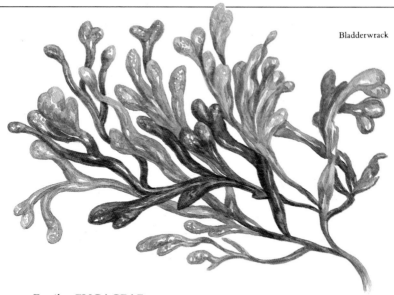

Bladderwrack

Family: FUCACEAE
Part used: Whole plant
Constituents and uses: This common seaweed provides a rich supply of a range of minerals, notably iodine. It is used to help stimulate activity in the thyroid gland. This gland produces a hormone which regulates the body's rate of energy use, the "tickover" rate of metabolism. It can help in problems of obesity, particularly if connected with an under-active thyroid gland.

In cases of rheumatism and arthritis, it can be taken as an infusion or in tablet form, as its mineral content makes it a popular nutritional supplement, or as a poultice over the affected areas.

Common name: BURDOCK
Botanical name: ARCTIUM LAPPA
Family: COMPOSITAE
Part used: Root
Constituents and uses: This is one of the main alternative remedies used for skin problems such as eczema and psoriasis, and localized infections such as boils and abscesses. It contains bitters, volatile oils and tannins and its main action is in stimulating the digestive organs and the eliminatory organs. It is an ingredient of the

well-known "dandelion and burdock" drink, which now made commercially, is only a soda drink. When made at home from the real dandelion and burdock roots, it would have an excellent "inner cleansing" action.

It can be taken as a decoction, 3 times daily, and is best made fairly weak initially, as it is very effective. It can produce the unpleasant symptoms of "toxic crisis" if taken in large doses. Toxic crisis refers to the condition when the symptoms seem to get worse before they start to get better.

Common name: CARAWAY
Botanical name: CARUM CARVI
Family: UMBELLIFERAE
Part used: Dried seeds
Constituents and uses: These aromatic seeds, with a high volatile oil content, are very soothing to the digestive system. They will ease colic and flatulence and the tannin content makes them a useful treatment for diarrhea.

The qualities of the volatile oil also help to ease chest congestion such as in bronchitis, and will help promote the production of breast milk in nursing mothers.

It makes a pleasant drink, as an infusion, taken 3 times a day.

Common name: CARDAMOM
Botanical name: ELETTARIA CARDAMOMUM
Family: ZINGIBERACEAE
Part used: Seeds
Constituents and uses: These large, pungently aromatic seeds contain a large amount of volatile oil. They help to stimulate a sluggish digestion, and will soothe any irritation that may cause colic or flatulence. Their main active constituent is a volatile oil. An infusion can be made from the seeds, which should be crushed to help release the oil.

Common name: CASCARA
Botanical name: RHAMNUS PURSHIANA
Family: RHAMNACEAE
Part used: Bark
Constituents and uses: **Cascara** is useful in conditions of long-term sluggish constipation. It is one of a group of remedies containing

substances known as anthraquinones which act by stimulating, to the point of irritation, the lining of the upper intestines; this produces a reflex activation of the muscles further along in the colon, which then results in a bowel motion. The drawback of this treatment is that the muscle can go into an over-active state, causing griping pains and colic. However, cascara is one of the gentler remedies in the group, and can be described as a general digestive/intestinal tonic. It also contains bitters, which contribute to its tonic effects, and tannins which help modify the strength of the laxative action. The bark is made into a decoction and taken at night to be effective the next morning. It may be combined with any of the carminative, anti-griping remedies for a more soothing – and palatable – drink.

Common name: CAYENNE
Alternative common names(s): CHILLIES
Botanical name: CAPSICUM MINIMUM
Family: SOLANACEAE
Part used: Fruits
Constituents and uses: The hottest spice available! This remedy must be used with care, as too much can be irritating to the stomach when taken internally. The action mirrors the taste – it has strong warming and stimulating actions on the digestion and the circulation, and is used when there is a weakness or deficiency in either system. Sluggish dyspepsia and flatulence will respond, plus all the circulatory problems that are worsened by cold weather. This remedy is also excellent for chills, generally, and respiratory problems that are associated with cold, damp weather. For internal use, a tea made with $^1/_8$ a teaspoon of crushed cayenne to 220ml (1 cup) of water should be taken three times a day. A pleasant compound mixture of circulatory stimulants known as "Composition Essence" is another very convenient way of taking cayenne. $^1/_4 - ^1/_2$ a teaspoon can be added to hot drinks. Externally, the tea can be added to a small amount of warm water and used as a hand or footbath, very useful for poor circulation and chilblains in cold weather. **Do not use** on broken skin – it will be very painful!

Common name: CELANDINE (GREATER)
Botanical name: CHELIDONIUM MAJUS

Family: PAPAVERACEAE
Part used: Fresh juice
Constituents and uses: This plant excels as a treatment for warts. The orange, milky sap, containing enzymes that break down the tissue of warts, should be applied 3 times a day and will be effective within 2 or 3 weeks. As the plant dies off in the winter, this treatment is limited to spring and summer only.

Common name: CELANDINE (LESSER)
Alternative common names(s): PILEWORT
Botanical name: RANUNCULUS FICARIA
Family: RANUNCULACEAE
Part used: Dried leaves and stems
Constituents and uses: This plant makes an excellent application to hemorrhoids. It has an astringent action which helps to shrink and tone the walls of the dilated blood vessels. A lotion can be made from a strong infusion (or ointments are available) to be applied as needed, initially 3 times daily.

CAUTION: **It is not recommended to be taken internally.**

Common name: CELERY
Botanical name: APIUM GRAVEOLENS
Family: UMBELLIFERAE
Part used: Seeds
Constituents and uses: **Celery seeds** have a beneficial action on the kidneys. They help to stimulate the removal of waste products from the body via the kidneys and promote the flow of urine to "flush through" the urinary system. Both of these actions are useful in arthritis, rheumatism and gout where the accumulation of acids in the body either triggers or irritates the condition.

The main constituent of the seeds is the characteristically scented volatile oil. This is also antiseptic to the urinary system, useful in the treatment of kidney infections and cystitis.

Celery is an excellent cleansing food, but the plant contains less of the active therapeutic constituents than the seeds. Take the seeds as an infusion, 3 times daily.

Common name: CHAMOMILE – GERMAN
Botanical name: MATRICARIA RECUTITA
Family: COMPOSITAE
Part used: Flowers
Constituents and uses: There are two kinds of **Chamomile** used medicinally. The **German Chamomile** is the most widely available and has very similar properties to the other, which is known as **Roman Chamomile**. Both have a similar scent, emitted from the oils in the plants.

The title "Mother of the Gut" suggests the respect in which **German Chamomile** is held. It is anti-inflammatory, and will help soothe gastric irritation, dyspepsia, flatulence and colic: it also has a bitter constituent which helps stimulate an underactive digestion. It has a gentle relaxing influence on the nervous system generally, and is particularly useful where nervous tension is affecting the digestive system. It may help women suffering from painful periods, and is useful in any problems with children where an over-excitable nature is causing difficulties.

It is taken as an infusion as required – it makes a pleasant alternative to ordinary tea. It can be obtained as an essential oil – a drop of this can be taken on a sugar cube or in honey. This can be diluted 1:20 with almond oil and used as an anti-inflammatory massage oil. Alternatively it can be added to a bowl of hot water and used as a steam inhalation for irritation and inflammation in the respiratory tract.

Common name: CHICKWEED
Botanical name: STELLARIA MEDIA
Family: CARYOPHYLLACEAE
Part used: Leaves: dried or fresh
Constituents and uses: This abundant weed can be eaten fresh, in sandwiches, and is a good source of iron. It is used for its therapeutic value as an anti-irritant when applied to the skin. It soothes and heals damaged skin, and reduces itching and irritation in rashes and eczema. It can be applied as a poultice, or obtained in an ointment base for use on small areas of skin.

If the affected area is large, a strong infusion can be added to the bath water to cover the whole surface of the body. The fresh plant, if available, should be used in preference to the dried form.

Common name: CINNAMON
Botanical name: CINNAMOMUM ZEYLANICUM
Family: LAURACEAE
Part used: Dried bark, sections of which become curled at the edges and thus known as "quills"
Constituents and uses: A most pleasant and gentle carminative, anti-griping, anti-flatulent remedy due to its volatile oils. It helps to prevent uncomfortable "bloating", is useful against nausea and, due to the tannins it contains, has a mild anti-diarrheal action.

Finely divided pieces of bark can be taken as an infusion. It can be added freely to other herbal preparations to improve the taste. It is best taken before or after meals to aid digestion.

Common name: CLEAVERS
Alternative common names(s): GOOSEGRASS
Botanical name: GALIUM APARINE
Family: RUBIACEAE
Part used: Leaves and stems
Constituents and uses: This plant helps stimulate the expulsion of fluid via the kidneys, so is useful for urinary problems. It is also one of the main remedies for treating problems associated with swelling of the lymph glands. These are frequently activated in localized infections and may be noticed as small hard swellings, such as in the neck in a case of tonsillitis (the tonsils themselves are lymphatic tissue). The lymph glands basically "trap" infections and prevent them from being passed to further areas of the body.

Cleavers

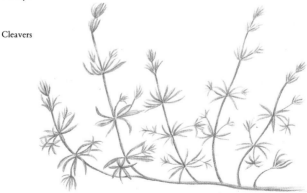

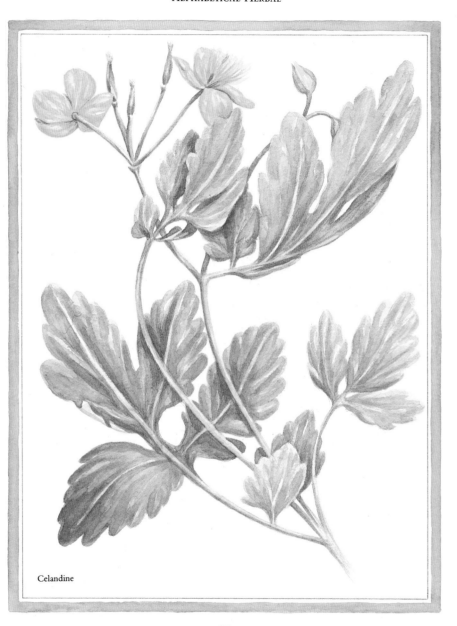

Celandine

In a long-term lymphatic disturbance, fluid retention may develop, and cleavers will be doubly useful then due to its diuretic properties. It is a good "cleansing" remedy generally and is applicable to a wide range of illnesses where this action is required.

It should be taken as an infusion, 3 times daily.

Common name: COLTSFOOT
Botanical name: TUSSILAGO FARFARA
Family: COMPOSITAE
Part used: Flowers and leaves
Constituents and uses: Unlike many of the expectorant remedies which have an irritating effect, **Coltsfoot** helps to ease the irritation and tightness connected with chest infections where there is particularly a dry, unproductive cough – typically the "barking" cough. This can be painful and persistent and responds better to **Coltsfoot** than practically any other remedy. Children who are kept awake at night by a persistent cough are usually greatly helped by it. It contains bitters, glycosides and a generous amount of the mineral zinc. It is thought that this may well contribute to the plant's beneficial properties as it seems to be vital in the body's defenses against infection.

An infusion of either the flowers or the leaves should be taken 3 times a day.

CAUTION: **Recent research has shown the presence of two alkaloids in the young flowers which when tested on rats caused liver cancer. Although these compounds exist in low concentrations in the flowers and leaves, any prolonged medical use is not advised. Coltsfoot is an ingredient of some herbal tobaccos. These should be avoided as should all smoking.**

Common name: COMFREY
Alternative common names(s): KNITBONE
Botanical name: SYMPHYTUM OFFICINALE
Family: BORAGINACEAE
Part used: Leaves and roots
Constituents and uses: **Comfrey** is the most useful of the healing remedies. Its constituents include astringent tannins, soothing mucilage, resin and a substance called allantoin. This has the

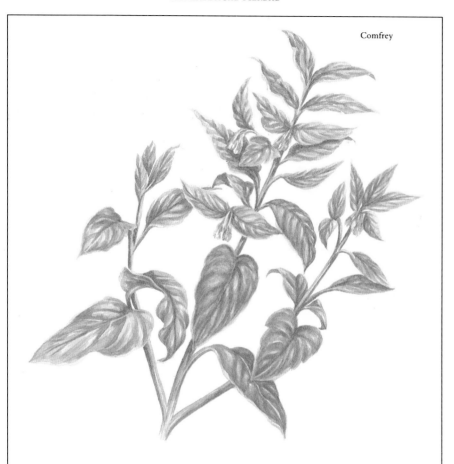

Comfrey

ability to stimulate the growth of new cells, by speeding up the rate at which DNA, the "blueprint" of the cell, is produced: after this stage, all other parts of the cell follow automatically.

The leaves can be taken internally for stomach and duodenal ulcers, where the tannins and mucilage help calm any inflammation; the allantoin will heal the eroded area. This remedy is also appropriate for chest problems such as bronchitis where it has a soothing and healing action.

Externally the root or leaves can be used as a poultice over any clean wound, or deeper problem such as tendon and ligament damage. Traditionally it has been used to heal broken bones – the root poultice dries to a very hard consistency, providing valuable support in the days before plaster casts were available.

The ointment can be used regularly in place of a poultice – it is a very useful part of every home's first-aid kit for minor injuries.

CAUTION: **Concern has been expressed over the safety of taking Comfrey internally, due to a constituent alkaloid which is known to be toxic. Experiments using the isolated alkaloid have shown it to be damaging to the liver. Although there has never been any evidence of the whole herb causing similar damage, I must advise caution in its use. If you are considering using the herb internally, contact a qualified herbalist for advice.**

At present, Comfrey is still legally available as a loose herb, but it may be withdrawn from licensed herbal medicines (those formulations that are available over the counter in health shops) in the future.

There are no restrictions on using Comfrey externally – it is totally safe when applied to the skin.

Common name: CUDWEED, MARSH
Botanical name: GNAPHALIUM ULIGINOSUM
Family: COMPOSITAE
Part used: Leaves and stems
Constituents and uses: This plant helps in nasal and throat catarrh. It is thought to contain small amounts of volatile oil and tannins which enhance its beneficial properties; it can be taken as an infusion, both as a gargle or as a drink, 3 times a day. Severe throat infections such as tonsillitis and quinsy usually respond well, but are best treated by **Cudweed** in combination with other astringent and anti-infective remedies.

Common name: DAMIANA
Botanical name: TURNERA DIFFUSA
Family: TURNERACEAE
Part used: Leaves and stems
Constituents and uses: This remedy is reputed to be a male aphrodisiac, though in my opinion there is no one simple medicinal solution to the range of problems that may cause

difficulties in sexual function. It has an action on the male reproductive system similar to that of the male hormone testosterone, which will enhance sexual function if the problems are of a purely physical nature. It certainly is of great benefit in nervous problems such as anxiety and depression. It has a combined tonic and almost nutritional effect on nerve tissue, due to the combination of constituents: bitters, tannins, resins, oils, and alkaloids, including caffeine. Both sexes will benefit from this action. It can be taken as an infusion 3 times daily.

Common name: DANDELION
Botanical name: TARAXACUM OFFICINALE
Family: COMPOSITAE
Part used: Leaves and root
Constituents and uses:

Leaves

One of the most useful diuretic remedies. It is particularly beneficial in fluid retention due to heart problems, as it contains a useful amount of the mineral potassium. This is vital for healthy function of the heart muscle, but is often lost via the urine when diuretic drugs are used. **Dandelion leaves**, with their natural content of potassium make up the loss automatically. They are also useful for other problems where the kidneys need to be stimulated, such as urinary infections or pre-menstrual fluid retention. Take an infusion 3 times daily.

Root

Dandelion root is a good liver stimulant. This makes it useful for a wide range of problems. It will improve the appetite and stimulate sluggish digestive functions due to its bitter properties. It helps in problems such as jaundice and gall-bladder disease. It also has a gentle laxative effect and will help the liver's detoxifying functions – useful in rheumatism and arthritis, or any other illness where a build-up of waste products is contributing to the problem. The liver is the main organ which has the job of eliminating alien substances, such as artificial additives in the food we eat, or airborne pollution such as chemical fumes.
Dandelion root will help support the health of people who are particularly susceptible to these substances.

Dandelion

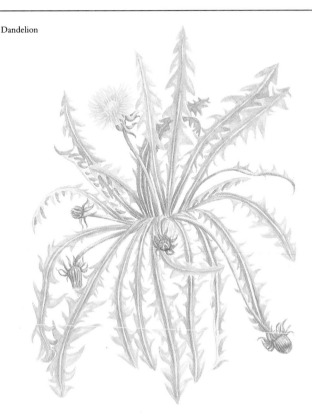

Common name: DEVIL'S CLAW
Botanical name: HARPAGOPHYTUM PROCUMBENS
Family: PEDALIACEAE
Part used: Tuber (underground stem)
Constituents and uses: Used in the treatment of arthritis, rheumatism and fibrositis, this plant contains glycosides which have an anti-inflammatory and possibly detoxifying action. It may help as a mild analgesic to relieve the pain of muscular and arthritic inflammation.

It should be taken as a decoction, 3 times daily, and is most likely to help when combined with other anti-arthritic and detoxifying remedies.

Common name: DOCK, YELLOW
Botanical name: RUMEX CRISPUS
Family: POLYGONACEAE
Part used: Root
Constituents and uses: This plant acts on the liver and intestines. It is useful for skin problems where the eliminative and detoxifying functions of the body need stimulation, such as eczema, acne and psoriasis. It contains bitters and laxative glycosides which stimulate muscular activity in the intestines. This, however, is reduced by the astringent action of tannins in the plant, so it has a gentle rather than severe action. It can also be used for liver and gall-bladder diseases.

A decoction should be taken 3 times daily.

Common name: ECHINACEA
Alternative common names(s): CONEFLOWER
Botanical name: ECHINACEA ANGUSTIFOLIA
Family: COMPOSITAE
Part used: Root
Constituents and uses: This is one of the main anti-infective remedies and is effective against viral, fungal and bacterial infections. It works in a twofold way: by destroying the harmful organisms directly and by stimulating the response of the body's immune system. It also has a cleansing "alterative" action and helps promote the body's series of activities by which the whole process of inflammation, as well as the infection, is healthily resolved. It can be used to help acute infections, such as tonsillitis, abscesses and boils, and longer lasting, entrenched problems such as bronchitis, pelvic infections and sinusitis.

A decoction should be taken 3 times daily.

Common name: ELDER
Botanical name: SAMBUCUS NIGRA
Family: CAPRIFOLIACEAE
Part used: Flowers and berries
Constituents and uses:
Flowers
The flowers contain a volatile oil that gives the characteristic scent, also a bio-flavonoid that helps to strengthen the walls of

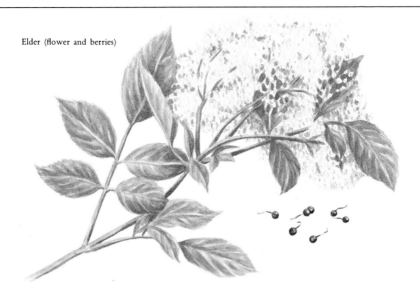

Elder (flower and berries)

damaged blood vessels. The main action of the flower is on the circulation – it helps to promote perspiration and is very useful when taken as a tea to ease a feverish cold or the flu. A second property is that it soothes the condition of inflamed nasal passages and helps relieve catarrh – I recommend it as a very pleasant drink for anyone who has long-term, hard-to-shift catarrh or sinusitis. However, it is not an anti-infective remedy and must be combined with one if there is an infection present.

Berries

Elderberry wine is a traditional remedy for rheumatic and arthritic problems; it has a mild laxative and diuretic effect.

Common name: ELECAMPANE
Botanical name: INULA HELENIUM
Family: COMPOSITAE
Part used: Root
Constituents and uses: Very useful in the treatment of chest infections. It has a soothing, expectorant action – due to its essential oils and mucilage – which helps to expel infected phlegm. It also has anti-infective properties and its component of bitters

Eyebright

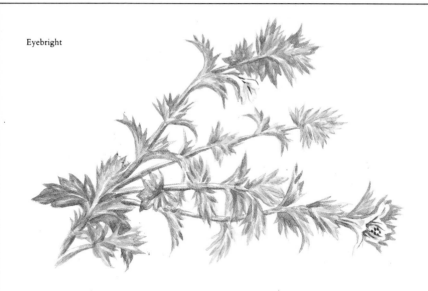

helps to stimulate the digestive system, thus dealing with any debility caused by the lung disease.

A decoction should be taken 3 times daily.

Common name: EYEBRIGHT
Botanical name: EUPHRASIA OFFICINALIS
Family: SCHROPHULARIACEAE
Part used: Leaves
Constituents and uses: As its name suggests, this plant has long been used as a topical application for eye irritations. It contains tannins, resins and volatile oil which have astringent and anti-inflammatory properties. These help problems due to allergic reactions, airborne pollution (for example, smoky atmospheres) and conjunctivitis.

When used as a gargle, it will help catarrhal and inflammatory problems of the throat and nose; take internally for the same.

For bathing the eyes, a half-strength infusion should be made and allowed to cool. This must be strained thoroughly – a paper coffee filter is suitable – then put in an eyebath and used to irrigate the whole surface of the eye. If there is an infection present the eyebath must be immersed in boiling water and the solution changed after use on the first eye. The strength of the infusion may be increased gradually, if this is necessary, to gain maximum benefit from the remedy. A gargle should be made from a full-strength infusion. This can be swallowed after gargling. **Eyebright** is best combined with an equal quantity of **Golden Seal** when used in an eyebath for eye infections.

Common name: FENNEL
Botanical name: FOENICULUM VULGARE
Family: UMBELLIFERAE
Part used: Seeds
Constituents and uses: This is another of the sweet, aromatic spices with a high volatile oil content. It also contains bitter substances, giving the duel benefit of stimulating a sluggish digestion and helping to calm the irritation that can result in griping pains, flatulence and over-activity in the bowel.

Like many of the aromatic spices, it helps stimulate milk production in lactating mothers.

An infusion of the seeds can be taken before or after meals to aid the digestion. This remedy is so well known as a pleasant herbal tea that it is easily available in the form of tea-bags.

Common name: FENUGREEK
Botanical name: TRIGONELLA FOENUM-GRAECUM
Family: LEGUMINOSEAE
Part used: Seeds
Constituents and uses: This pungently aromatic bitter-tasting spice contains a variety of constituents which help the digestion: bitters, mucilage and volatile oils, plus an anti-inflammatory steroid-like substance which further helps to calm conditions such as gastritis and enteritis. It has a tonic effect on the digestion, particularly for convalescents.

Its anti-inflammatory properties will help when it is applied as a poultice to inflamed or infected skin.

The steroid component, as well as the oils, helps stimulate milk production in lactating mothers.

An infusion of the seeds should be taken before or after meals, in combination with other sweet aromatic spices which will improve the taste. A poultice is made from the crushed seeds.

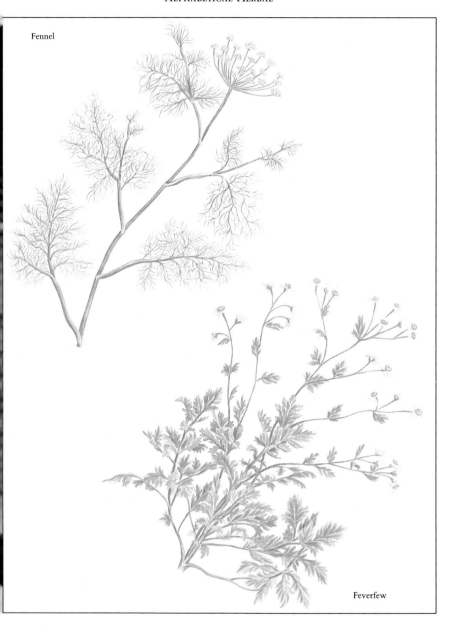

Fennel

Feverfew

Common name: FEVERFEW
Botanical name: TANACETUM PARTHENIUM
Family: COMPOSITAE
Part used: Leaves
Constituents and uses: This remedy has two different, equally useful applications. It has been tested in migraine clinics and found to be successful in about seventy percent of migraine cases – achieving at least partial improvement and often total remission of the problem. It helps to open up the constricted blood-vessels in the brain that cause the pain in the majority of migraine cases. It contains volatile oil and tannin.

The anti-arthritic properties were discovered when migraine sufferers taking **Feverfew** found that their arthritis was also improving. It is one of the few anti-inflammatory remedies that is likely to bring about an improvement when taken by itself rather than in combination with other remedies – other anti-inflammatory herbs may help improve the condition in other ways.

It is best taken in the spring and summer as freshly picked leaves – one or two large leaves daily should be put in a sandwich (to mask the bitter taste, and the possible irritating effects on the mouth). The plant dies off in the winter. Capsules containing the freeze-dried leaves are available, alternatively the dried leaves can be taken as an infusion.

Common name: GARLIC
Botanical name: ALLIUM SATIVUM
Family: LILLICEAE
Part used: "Clove" – in botanical terms, a corm
Constituents and uses: This plant is best known for its culinary properties, but is highly beneficial as preventative medicine when taken regularly. An important point, however, is that to retain its greatest benefit, it must be eaten **raw** – cooking destroys most of its therapeutic properties. It contains a high amount of volatile oil and when the clove is crushed, certain constituents in this interact to produce the characteristically odored, actively antiseptic principle of the plant. This is of great benefit in the treatment of infections in the digestive tract, and has the remarkable ability to act selectively against harmful micro-organisms here, while leav-

ing intact the beneficial bacterial populations which aid the digestive process.

As the constituents are absorbed into the bloodstream and dispersed around the body, the antiseptic principles, when passing through the blood vessels in the lungs, diffuse out through the lung membranes and are "breathed out" of the body. The remedy is therefore excellent against respiratory infections – both deep in the lungs and throat and higher up in the nasal passages or sinuses. This explains why the smell of **Garlic** is so persistent – it is due to the way that it comes out of the body, rather than how it goes in.

The second great benefit of the plant is its importance as an aid to circulatory problems. It contains a "healing" mineral called germanium and a group of substances which help to control fat levels in the bloodstream – an important action, as fat deposition is a great problem in hardening of the arteries, angina, and many cases of high blood pressure. It also helps to prevent thrombosis by counteracting the tendency of clot-forming cells to stick together within the blood vessels.

Up to one clove of fresh raw **Garlic** should be taken daily, in divided doses, for the benefit of one's general health. If the taste is found to be really unacceptable, **Garlic Oil** capsules can be substituted – 2 or 3, if taken at night, will have passed out of the body by the following morning.

Common name: GINGER
Botanical name: ZINGIBERIS OFFICINALE
Family: ZINGIBERACEAE
Part used: Root
Constituents and uses: One of the strongest of the aromatic remedies. It contains volatile oils and phenols and has a strong stimulant action on the digestion and circulation. It helps to calm flatulence and colic but, although less hot than cayenne, is best initially given in small doses, as it can be irritating to the stomach in large doses. One recently discovered benefit is the ease it brings to sufferers of travel sickness – it seems to have a directly soothing effect to prevent vomiting and dizziness.

It has a warming, anti-chilling effect on the whole circulation, promoting blood flow to the extremities, and is useful internally

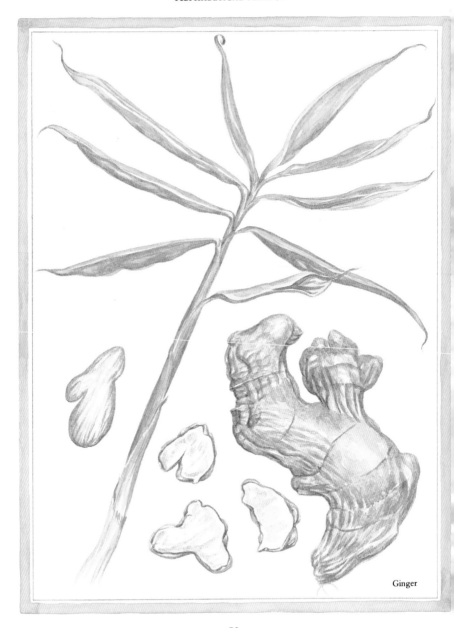

Ginger

and locally for problems related to poor circulation due to cold weather, typically chilblains.

Make an infusion of the finely sliced fresh root of a strength to suit individual taste. Alternatively, use well-preserved powdered ginger – it should still have the characteristic aromatic scent.

For travel sickness, a small piece of crystallized ginger can be taken, before starting and throughout the journey.

For hand and footbaths, a strong infusion should be made and added to a bowl of warm water. Immerse the hands or feet for about 5–10 minutes. If the bath causes stinging on any broken skin, add more water until an acceptable dilution is reached.

Common name: GOLDEN ROD
Botanical name: SOLIDAGO VIRGAUREA
Family: COMPOSITAE
Part used: Leaves
Constituents and uses: A useful remedy for catarrhal problems. It contains tannins, bitters, oils, soap-like substances known as saponins and a sugar-related glycoside. It has an anti-inflammatory and anti-infective action, and helps particularly with long-term nasal catarrh where the infection may be stubborn, if low-grade.

Take an infusion 3 times daily, and combine with other anti-catarrhal and cleansing remedies for best results.

Common name: GOLDEN SEAL
Botanical name: HYDRASTIS CANADENSIS
Family: RANUCULACEAE
Part used: Root – botanically a rhizome
Constituents and uses: **Golden Seal** contains oils, resin and several substances known as alkaloids which give it much of its characteristic action. It is used as a tonic to all mucous membranes, particularly of the digestive system, where it has a stimulating and laxative action. It helps to stimulate liver, kidney and lung function and it is an antiseptic remedy in mouth, ear and eye infections.

Make a decoction, or an infusion from the powered root, to take 3 times daily. An infusion, strained through a filter paper, can be used as a gargle for mouth and throat infections. This can be

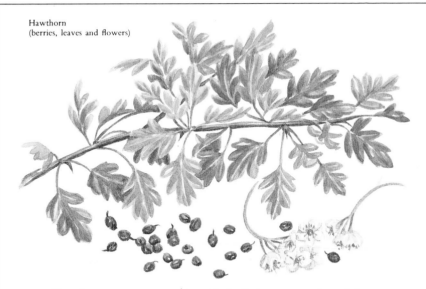

Hawthorn
(berries, leaves and flowers)

diluted to quarter strength with boiled water and used in an eyebath for eye infections – it is best combined with **Eyebright**. CAUTION: **This is one of the few remedies that should be avoided until the last month of pregnancy, as it may stimulate contractions in the muscle of the womb.**

Common name: HAWTHORN
Alternative common names(s): MAY TREE
Botanical name: CRATAEGUS OXYACANTHOIDES
Family: ROSACEAE
Part used: Berries, leaves and flowers
Constituents and uses: A remedy of great benefit to many problems of the heart and blood vessels. It contains several bio-flavonoids (which are a source of nutrition to the heart and blood vessels), tannins, glycosides and saponins. Hawthorn helps to "feed" and strengthen the heart muscle; it opens up the heart's own supply of blood and stabilizes and strengthens the beat. It is therefore useful in all types of heart failure and debility, including angina, and as a preventative treatment for heart attacks, plus as a restorative after they have occurred. It helps to reduce high blood pressure, and, paradoxically, can be used in cases of low blood

pressure as it seems to have an overall normalizing action. It is useful in cases of hardening of the arteries and in any other illnesses where the problem originates in the blood vessels, such as varicose veins and inflammation of the blood vessels.

My personal preference is to take this remedy in the form of berries, crushed and made into an infusion, 3 times daily.

Common name: HOPS
Botanical name: HUMULUS LUPULUS
Family: CANNABINACEAE
Part used: Strobiles – the fruiting-body which appears after flowering
Constituents and uses: The papery strobiles contain resins, bitters and tannins. Originally used in ale to enhance its preservation properties.

It has two main uses in modern herbal medicine: the stimulating effect of its bitter properties on the digestion; and its soothing and relaxing effects on the muscular activity of the digestive system and on the nervous system generally. It is useful in the treatment of colic, colitis and irritable bowel (which is often linked to nervous tension), plus general nervous tension and insomnia.

Hops

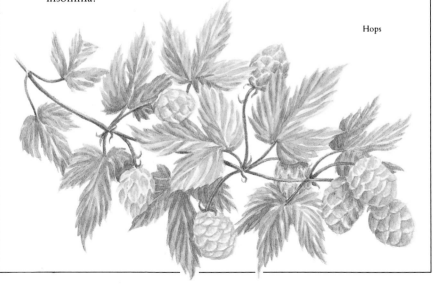

Make an infusion – initially weak due to the strength of the taste – to take 3 times daily or at night. A traditional way of bringing about restful sleep is with the use of a hop pillow – simply a small pillow-shaped cotton bag, filled with dried hops.

CAUTION: **Due to the effectiveness of its relaxing, sedative properties, it should not be used in cases of depression – it may worsen rather than relieve this problem.**

Common name: HOREHOUND (WHITE)
Botanical name: MARRUBIUM VULGARE
Family: LABIATAE
Part used: Leaves
Constituents and uses: This is a gentle but effective soothing expectorant. It helps to relax tightness and encourages the production and expulsion of phlegm from the lungs. It contains mucilage, tannins, volatile oil and bitter substances which help the digestion and liver function. It is very useful in all chest infections, particularly where there is a dry, unproductive cough and associated poor appetite and debility in the digestive system.

An infusion should be taken 3 times daily.

Common name: HORSETAIL
Botanical name: EQUISETUM ARVENSE
Family: EQUISETACEAE

Horsetail

Part used: Aerial parts – is too primitive to have true leaves
Constituents and uses: An excellent remedy for urinary problems, this plant is a soothing, healing diuretic. It contains numerous minerals, including silica, which may be significant in its healing action. It also has bitters, flavonoids, saponins and alkaloids. It promotes the expulsion of fluid through the urinary system and helps soothe any inflammation there may be, whether due to infection or other causes. It tones and heals further damage, and can be used for prostate disease. It has a good reputation as a treatment for bed-wetting in children, though this problem is rarely just a physical problem, in my opinion: **Horsetail** may play a useful part, rather than solve the problem entirely.

An infusion should be taken 3 times daily.

Common name: HYSSOP
Botanical name: HYSSOPUS OFFICINALIS
Family: LABIATAE
Part used: Leaves and flowers together
Constituents and uses: One of the remedies used to help the treatment of the common cold. It helps in respiratory infections, as an expectorant for chest problems, and as an anti-catarrhal in head colds and sinusitis. It encourages sweating, and is therefore useful in the early stages of a feverish infection. It also has a soothing influence on the nervous system, allaying tension and anxiety. It has been used in cases of *petit mal*, which is a minor form of epilepsy.

Take an infusion 3 times daily. If the head cold is proving particularly debilitating, take the infusion more frequently – up to every 2 hours – in combination with the other cold remedies.

Common name: LAVENDER
Botanical name: LAVANDULA OFFICINALIS
Family: LABIATAE
Part used: Flowers
Constituents and uses: It may come as a surprise that this plant, so well known as a scent, is also used medicinally. The volatile oil that gives off the scent also gives the flowers their medicinal qualities: as a gentle, soothing tonic for the nervous system and digestive system. **Lavender** helps in cases of nervous anxiety and

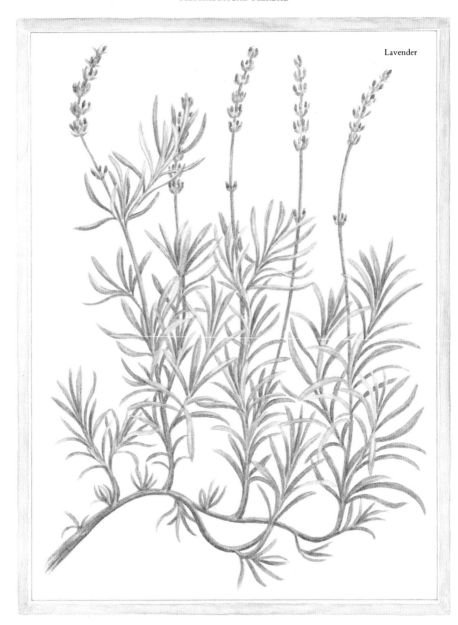

Lavender

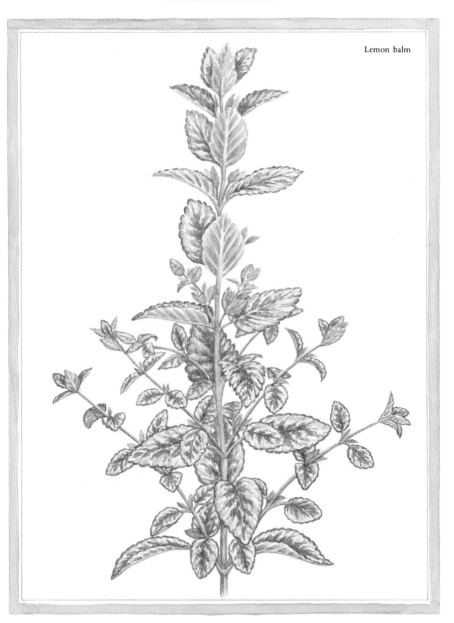

Lemon balm

debility, exhaustion and depression. It may relieve tension head-aches and help to soothe digestive flatulence and colic.

An infusion should be taken 3 times daily, before or after meals to help the digestion.

Common name: LEMON BALM
Alternative common names(s): BALM
Botanical name: MELISSA OFFICINALIS
Family: LABIATAE
Part used: Leaves
Constituents and uses: A relaxing remedy for the nervous and digestive systems. The pleasant lemony scent comes from the volatile oil in the plant, which also contains bitters and tannins. It is used in the treatment of nervous dyspepsia, indigestion, colic and flatulence. It will also help where the nervous symptoms are prominent in themselves, such as anxiety and nervous tension.

An infusion should be taken 3 times daily, and can be enjoyed as a pleasant drink.

Common name: LIMEFLOWERS
Botanical name: TILIA CORDATA or PLATYPHYLLOS
Family: TILIACEAE
Part used: Flowers and leaf-like bract
Constituents and uses: The lime is a well-known tree, scenting the air when flowering in July. This scent will be recognized as the same as in **Limeflower tea**. The flowers contain volatile oils, tannins, mucilage, saponins and flavonoids, and the main actions are on the nervous and circulatory systems. It is a gentle relaxing remedy, soothing anxiety and tension and aiding sleep when taken at night. It is a favorite remedy for tension, restlessness and over-excitability in children. It can be used with confidence to combat any childhood illness where these characteristics are contributing to the overall problem.

It helps to open up the circulation of blood to the skin, which will encourage perspiration in cases of feverishness. It will also reduce high blood pressure by reducing tension in the muscle layer of the blood vessels. It is one of the few remedies reputed to have a healing effect on damaged linings in blood vessels.

An infusion can be taken 3 times daily, or at night to promote restful sleep. For infants, if the infusion is not to be taken by mouth, it can be added to the bath water and they will absorb it through their skin. It is a successful method of calming tired, fractious babies.

Common name: LICORICE
Botanical name: GLYCYRRHIZA GLABRA
Family: LEGUMINOSAE
Part used: Root
Constituents and uses: This plant contains a range of substances including glycosides, saponins, bitters, oils, tannins and flavonoids. It has a strong stimulating action on the adrenal glands, similar to the body's natural hormone for this function. An increase in adrenal steroid hormones results in an anti-inflammatory action on conditions such as arthritis and rheumatism.

It helps in chest infections, as a soothing expectorant. It is useful in the treatment of gastric ulcers as it forms a coating of thick, protective mucilage over the site of the ulcer. It also has a mild laxative effect on the lower digestive tract.

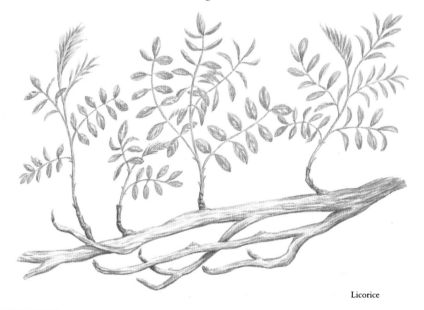

Licorice

A decoction should be taken 3 times a day. The root is also available to chew as a "sweetie".

CAUTION: **Due to the steroid-like action of the plant, it is not recommended to be taken in cases of high blood pressure.**

Common name: MARIGOLD
Alternative common name(s): ENGLISH POT MARIGOLD
Botanical name: CALENDULA OFFICINALIS
Family: COMPOSITAE
Part used: Flowers
Constituents and uses: This remedy is an invaluable antiseptic and healer. It contains bitters, oils and resins. It works well against fungal infections, and is particularly useful for the athlete's foot/thrush-type infections that affect skin and mucous membranes. It has a toning, anti-inflammatory and healing influence when applied topically to most skin problems, such as slow-healing wounds and minor burns and scalds; it is worth trying in cases of eczema and psoriasis. It is also beneficial as a local application to varicose veins and hemorrhoids. Internally, it is used in the treatment of gastric and duodenal ulcers.

An infusion should be taken internally 3 times daily. A double-strength infusion can be used as a lotion to apply to skin problems. Alternatively, a very convenient form of local application is marigold cream or ointment.

Common name: MARSHMALLOW
Botanical name: ALTHAEA OFFICINALIS
Family: MALVACEAE
Part used: ·Root and leaf
Constituents and uses: The root is one of the best sources of soothing mucilage, combined with anti-inflammatory tannins. It will help protect and soothe irritated mucous membranes. It has a very soothing influence on stomach inflammation and ulcers, and calms enteritis and colitis.

The leaves contain volatile oil, and are used in the treatment of dry, harsh coughs, to soothe and promote the expulsion of phlegm from the lungs. They also soothe the urinary system in cases of infection, and irritation from kidney or bladder stones.

The leaves can be taken as an infusion. The root is made into

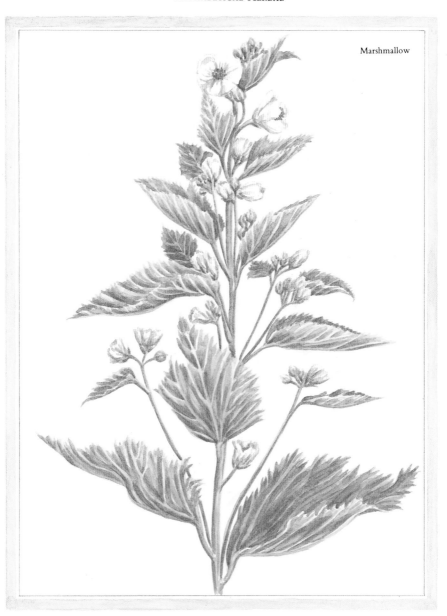

Marshmallow

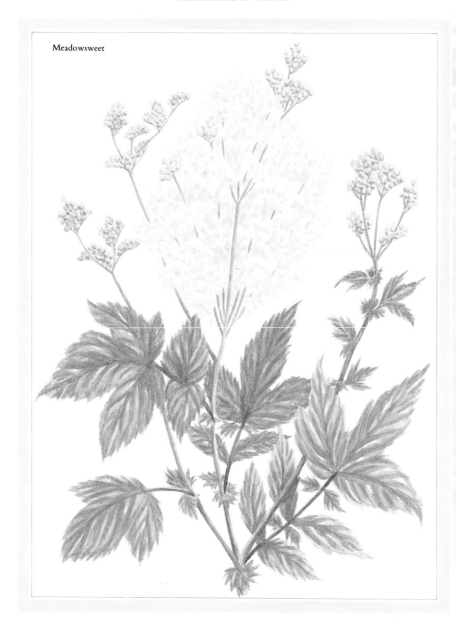

Meadowsweet

a very mucilaginous decoction. This can be used as a poultice on skin inflammation if made stronger, i.e., having a more mucilaginous almost paste-like consistency.

Common name: MEADOWSWEET
Botanical name: FILIPENDULA ULMARIA
Family: ROSACEAE
Part used: Leaves
Constituents and uses: This plant is most useful for its anti-acidic and anti-inflammatory properties. It contains volatile oil, tannins, is rich in minerals, and is a natural source of salicylic acid (aspirin). It has all the anti-inflammatory, anti-fever benefits of aspirin, without the side effects of stomach irritation. This is because the other constituents of the plant have an outstandingly beneficial action on stomach problems. It is most useful in problems of excess acidity and indigestion, heartburn, and stomach and duodenal ulcers.

Meadowsweet is also a useful anti-acidic and anti-inflammatory remedy in the treatment of rheumatism and arthritis. The flowers are gently astringent and are used for diarrhea in children. An infusion should be taken 3 times daily.

Common name: MOTHERWORT
Botanical name: LEONURUS CARDIACA
Family: LABIATAE
Part used: Leaves
Constituents and uses: Used for centuries as a tonic to the female reproductive system, this remedy, containing bitters, volatile oil, tannins and alkaloids, is a good basis for all prescriptions to help irregular menstrual cycles, painful periods, and pre-menstrual tension. It will help to allay anxiety and tension connected with most menstrual disorders. It is useful as an ingredient of a mixture taken in the last month of pregnancy, to prepare for labor. It can also be taken after birth to help the womb return to its normal shape and size, and to ease tension and anxiety.

As the botanical name suggests, it has a feeding, strengthening action on the heart, and can be used in all conditions where this would be helpful, such as high blood pressure, after heart attacks, and for hardening of the arteries. Take an infusion 3 times daily.

Common name: MYRRH
Botanical name: COMMIPHORA MOLMOL
Family: BURSERACEAE
Part used: Resin (dried gum)
Constituents and uses: This remedy has been prized for thousands of years for its anti-microbial properties. It contains bitters, oils, gums and resins. It has a very "antiseptic" smell and taste. It works in a twofold way: first, it has a direct action to destroy bacteria that comes into contact with it, and second, it helps stimulate the body's natural immune powers – the white cells of the blood.

Use as a gargle for mouth problems: aphthous ulcers, gingivitis, abscesses, tonsillitis, etc. Externally, apply to skin infections – spots, boils, abscesses, and early stages of cold sores.

The resin does not dissolve well in water, so the most effective and convenient preparation is the alcoholic tincture. This should be diluted – use about $1/2$ a teaspoon of the tincture to 3 tablespoons of warm water as a gargle. Sip after gargling in order that the immune system can benefit.

Apply to skin infections at the same dilution or more dilute, if it stings, on broken skin. Use full strength on unbroken skin.

Common name: NETTLES (STINGING)
Botanical name: URTICA DIOICA
Family: URTICACEAE
Part used: Leaves
Constituents and uses: **Nettles** are a rich source of iron and Vitamin C, and make a pleasant nourishing vegetable when picked young and tender and then cooked like spinach. Medicinally, they have a cleansing action on the body, helping to improve kidney function and the circulation. They have an astringent action and help stimulate the pancreas in the control of blood-sugar levels; they also promote milk flow in lactating mothers. **Nettles** are most commonly used in the treatment of skin disease, such as eczema and psoriasis, and to help circulation to the scalp to promote healthy hair growth.

An infusion should be taken 3 times daily. A strong infusion can be used, in combination with **Rosemary**, as a hair rinse, or as a lotion applied daily to improve hair and scalp condition.

Common name: OREGON GRAPE
Botanical name: MAHONIA AQUIFOLIUM
Family: BERBERIDACEAE
Part used: Root
Constituents and uses: This contains a range of alkaloids to stimulate the liver, having a gentle laxative and tonic cleansing action. It is useful in skin problems such as eczema and psoriasis, and other conditions where sluggish liver and digestive functions are involved. It may also help to allay nausea. Best used in combination with other "alternative" remedies for skin problems.

A decoction should be taken 3 times daily.

Common name: PASSIONFLOWER – generally referred to by its botanical name.
Botanical name: PASSIFLORA INCARNATA
Family: PASSIFLORACEAE
Part used: Leaves
Constituents and uses: One of the most reliable, relaxing herbs, this plant contains alkaloids which calm the nervous system. It is particularly useful for relieving muscle tension due to anxiety, and is a good remedy for nervous insomnia.

Occasionally it seems to cause sleepiness if taken during the day, in certain susceptible individuals, but generally this is not a problem. An infusion should be taken 3 times daily, or at night.

CAUTION: **It should be avoided in pregnancy due to its possible stimulating effect on the muscles of the womb.**

Common name: PEPPERMINT
Botanical name: MENTHA PIPERITA
Family: LABIATAE
Part used: Leaves
Constituents and uses: This well-known plant, as well as making a delicious drink, is beneficial for the digestion. The main active ingredient is the volatile oil, but the plant also contains bitters and tannins to help its action. It helps to soothe the digestive system, to allay nausea, to reduce colic and flatulence in the bowel, and is effective in conditions as severe as colitis. It is also useful in the feverish stage of colds and flu, as it promotes perspiration and

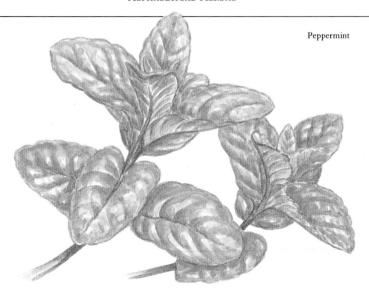

Peppermint

brings down the body temperature by opening up blood flow to the skin.

An infusion should be taken before or after meals to aid the digestion, or whenever a pleasant-tasting alternative drink to ordinary tea is required.

Common name: PSYLLIUM
Alternative common name(s): FLEA-SEED, ISPAGHULA
Botanical name: PLANTAGO PSYLLIUM
Family: PLANTAGINACEAE
Part used: Seeds
Constituents and uses: The dried seeds are surrounded with a cellulose coat, which swells to become a mucilaginous gel after being soaked in water. This provides an excellent bulking, lubricating, non-irritant laxative which helps all food through the digestive system more easily. It makes up for lack of fiber in the diet, without having the irritating effects on the sensitive lining of the digestive system caused by some high-fiber diets.

One or two teaspoons should be soaked in half a tumbler of water, or fruit juice to make it more palatable, for at least 4 hours or preferably overnight. Judge the amount needed according to results, which should be an easy motion within about 24 hours. This remedy is quite safe to take for an extended period of time, or as a regular part of the diet.

Common name: RASPBERRY LEAVES
Botanical name: RUBUS IDAEUS
Family: ROSACEAE
Part used: Leaves
Constituents and uses: This tannin-containing remedy has a soothing, astringent action, that is very useful for inflamed, sore throats. It should be sipped slowly to get the maximum benefit.

It is also beneficial for the female reproductive system – it can be taken before and during menstruation to ease discomfort and improve the efficiency of the muscle of the womb: similarly, in the last month or two of pregnancy it will help to tone the womb in preparation for labor and birth. It may assist during the week after the birth to help the womb return to its normal condition.

An infusion should be taken 3 times daily.

CAUTION: **It should not be taken during pregnancy, until the last 2 months, because of its possible muscle-stimulating effects.**

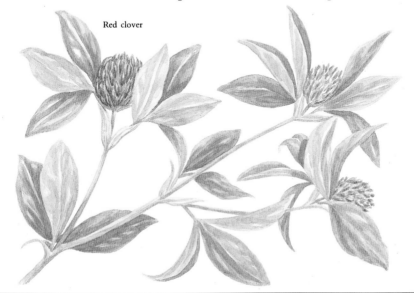

Red clover

Common name: RED CLOVER
Botanical name: TRIFOLIUM PRATENSE
Family: PAPILIONACEAE
Part used: Flowers
Constituents and uses: Most useful in childhood skin problems particularly eczema, it has a "cleansing" action through the kidneys. It helps loosen phlegm in the lungs, and may also have a slight anti-inflammatory action. It can be given to children with complete confidence.

An infusion should be taken 3 times daily.

Common name: RED SAGE
Botanical name: SALVIA OFFICINALIS
Family: LABIATAE
Part used: Leaves
Constituents and uses: A most useful soothing, healing and antiseptic remedy for throat and mouth infections. It contains a volatile oil, resin, tannins, saponins and flavonoids which may all contribute to its healing action. It can be used as a gargle, or taken

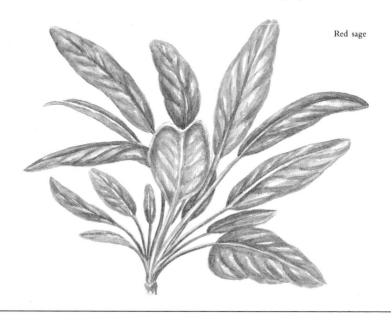

Red sage

internally – when it becomes an efficient anti-flatulent remedy. Its other main property is to reduce the secretions of the sweat and milk-producing glands, so it has a useful action against excessive perspiration. **Red Sage** can be taken by lactating mothers who are producing too much breastmilk, or when breast-feeding is being withdrawn.

Take an infusion as a gargle or sipped, 3 times daily.

CAUTION: **Avoid during pregnancy as it may have a stimulating effect on the muscle of the womb.**

Common name: ROSEMARY
Botanical name: ROSMARINUS OFFICINALIS
Family: LABIATAE
Part used: Leaves and stems
Constituents and uses: This plant has several uses; it contains oils, tannins, bitters and resin. It helps as a tonic to the liver and circulation, and has a relaxing, restorative effect on the nervous system. It can be used for nervous anxiety and tension and general debility after long-term nervous or physical illness. It helps relieve tension headaches and may be useful in migraine treatments.

Externally, apply to help dandruff and poor hair growth.

An infusion should be taken 3 times daily. A strong infusion can be used as a daily application to the scalp, or in hair-rinsing water to maintain the good condition of the hair.

Common name: SENNA
Alternative common names(s): ALEXANDRIA or TINNEVELLY SENNA
Botanical name: CASSIA ACUTIFOLA or ANGUSTIFOLIA
Family: LEGUMINOSAE
Part used: Fruits – known as "pods"
Constituents and uses: Probably the best-known herbal remedy! This laxative acts by irritating the lining of the upper intestines, which provokes reflex muscular activity in the colon, resulting in a bowel motion. The degree of irritation may also produce griping pains, so **Senna** is best taken with anti-griping remedies such as **Ginger, Cinnamon** or **Fennel**. It is best used only in the

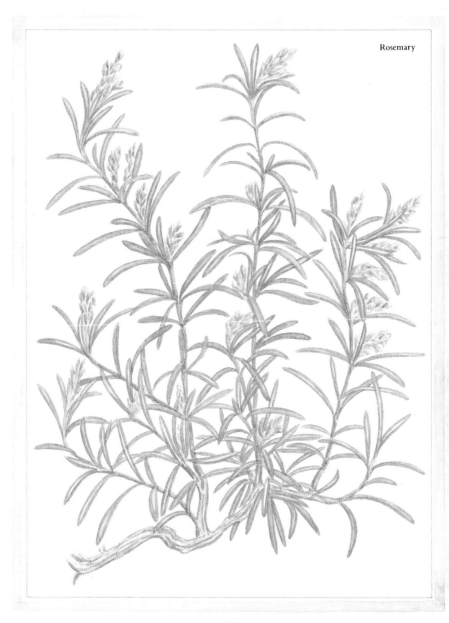

Rosemary

short-term, and for occasional rather than regular use.

Soak 3–6 Alexandrian pods, double Tinnevelly pods, in warm water for 8 hours; take at night for effect the following morning.

CAUTION: **Do not use in cases where colic or spastic colon are already features of the bowel disturbance.**

Common name: SLIPPERY ELM
Botanical name: ULMUS FULVA
Family: ULMACEAE
Part used: Powdered inner bark
Constituents and uses: The remedy most widely applicable to all digestive problems. It contains astringent tannins, but most of the benefit is due to the mucilage in the bark. When the powder is mixed with liquid it forms a gel consistency, which, when swallowed, puts a protective mucilaginous lining over the esophagus and stomach. This helps directly with an anti-inflammatory and calming action and it allows underlying healing to progress. It is very soothing after the discomfort of vomiting, and will help reduced irritation and over-activity in the bowel, via a nerve reflex action, as the stomach lining is soothed. It also works as a gentle bulking laxative remedy.

Take as often as required for stomach problems: add 1 teaspoon of the powder to a little cold milk, water or juice. When mixed to form a smooth paste, top up with warm liquid, stirring constantly. The consistency can be varied to suit individual taste.

Common name: ST. JOHN'S WORT
Botanical name: HYPERICUM PERFORATUM
Family: HYPERICACEAE
Part used: Leaves and flowers combined
Constituents and uses: When taken internally, this plant has a gentle relaxing and restorative action on the nervous system. It is used in cases of long-term nervous debility and fatigue and certain menopausal problems where anxiety is pronounced.

Externally, it is used to heal damaged skin; on cuts, grazes, bruises, minor burns, etc. It also has mild analgesic properties and may help to ease the pain of rheumatism, neuralgia and sciatica.

Take an infusion 3 times daily, or apply a poultice to affected

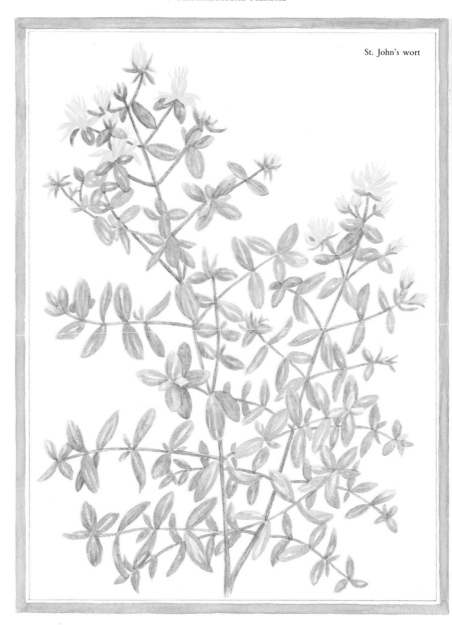

St. John's wort

areas. A cream or infused oil are also available – both very convenient forms of application.

Common name: THYME, COMMON
Botanical name: THYMUS VULGARIS
Family: LABIATAE
Part used: Leaves and flowers together
Constituents and uses: This well-loved garden shrub has antiseptic and expectorant properties. It contains a volatile oil, bitters, tannins, saponins and flavonoids. The antiseptic properties are most helpful to respiratory problems – used as a mouthwash or gargle, it will help mouth, gum and throat infections, and when taken internally it helps combat chest infections. It will loosen tight phlegm and thus ease a dry, barking cough.

Thyme will act as an anti-flatulent digestive tonic, and the tannins help against irritation and diarrhea.

An infusion should be taken 3 times daily. A strong infusion can be used as a mouthwash or gargle, 2 or 3 times daily.

Common name: VALERIAN
Botanical name: VALERIANA OFFICINALIS
Family: VALERIANACEAE
Part used: Root
Constituents and uses: The volatile oil in this plant gives it the characteristic smell that cats love! It also contains resins and gums and on humans it has a relaxing, calming action. It can be used for all types of nervous tension, anxiety, insomnia, etc., and will help to relax the muscle tension that may cause cramp, or colic if in the digestive system. It is very useful for reducing high blood pressure, particularly if nervous tension is one of the causes. Make a decoction of the root, to take 3 times daily.
CAUTION: **Occasionally, when taken in large amounts, it may have a stimulating rather than a relaxing effect.**

Common name: VERVAIN
Botanical name: VERBENA OFFICINALIS
Family: VERBENACEAE
Part used: Leaves and stems
Constituents and uses: This plant helps the nervous and digestive system. It contains bitters, tannins, volatile oil, glycosides, and an

Thyme

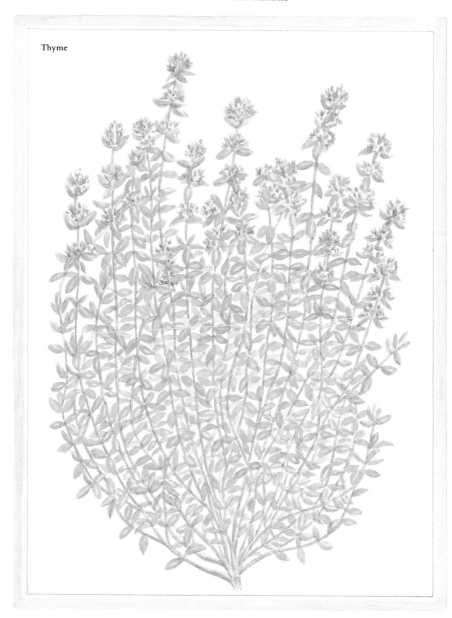

alkaloid. It is a restorative remedy for nervous exhaustion and debility, so is useful for physical and emotional/mental problems that effect the nervous system. It acts as a relaxant in cases of muscle tension and it is of great benefit in convalescent states. Its bitter tonic properties help stimulate the digestion and particularly liver function.

An infusion should be taken 3 times daily.

Common name: WHITE WILLOW
Botanical name: SALIX ALBA
Family: SALICACEAE
Part used: Bark
Constituents and uses: The name of salicylic acid (aspirin) was derived from the botanical name of the willow family: this plant is a good natural source of a similar substance. Taken in the natural form, side effects are less likely than when taking artificial aspirin. The benefits, however are similar: **White Willow** is used for its anti-inflammatory, anti-fever and mild analgesic properties. It is used in the treatment of rheumatism and arthritis to reduce pain and inflammation. It will help bring down a dangerously high temperature. It also contains tannins, which help to reduce inflammation in the digestive system.

A weak decoction should be taken 3 times daily, and is most effective when combined with other anti-rheumatic remedies, ideally **Meadowsweet.**

Common name: WILD LETTUCE
Botanical name: LACTUCA VIROSA
Family: COMPOSITAE
Part used: Leaves
Constituents and uses: This forerunner of the vegetable lettuce contains bitters and an alkaloid, and has a strong relaxing/sedative action. It is used to combat nervous tension, insomnia and over-excitability. It has a mild analgesic action, and may help to allay the pain of rheumatism, neuralgia, and menstrual cramps. The bitters exert a tonic action on the digestive organs.

An infusion should be taken 3 times daily.

NOTE: **The vegetable lettuce has a much milder action – one would have to eat two whole lettuces to notice the effect!**

Common name: WITCH HAZEL
Botanical name: HAMAMELIS VIRGINIANA
Family: HAMAMELIDACEAE
Part used: Bark, twigs, leaves
Constituents and uses: Best known in the clear liquid form, **Distilled Witch Hazel.** This should occupy a place in every first-aid box. The main constituents are tannins, though there is also a volatile oil and bitters. Externally the remedy is anti-inflammatory, soothing and cooling, and is very useful for any minor injury. It will ease bruises and swellings and will help staunch blood flow from small wounds: it also allays the discomfort of varicose veins and hemorrhoids. The distilled preparation should not be taken internally, but an infusion of the leaves can be made to soothe digestive problems where irritation and mucus discharge is present.
It should be taken 3 times daily.

Common name: YARROW
Alternative common name(s): MILFOIL
Botanical name: ACHILLEA MILLEFOLIUM
Family: UMBELLIFERAE
Part used: Leaves
Constituents and uses: This plant has a wide range of constituents, including oils, bitters, tannins, resins and salicylates. Its main action is on the circulation: it helps to improve circulation to the skin by opening up the surface blood vessels. This action promotes perspiration and is very useful in helping to control dangerously high temperatures. It also results in a lowering of blood pressure, and helps to improve the condition of damaged blood vessels. **Yarrow** is also useful in cases of varicose veins.
It can stimulate the appetite and aid the digestion. Its astringent properties may be useful, when taken internally, for heavy menstrual blood loss, and when applied externally it will help staunch the flow of blood from wounds. It has a good reputation as a healing agent in the treatment of slow and stubborn wounds.
An infusion should be taken 3 times daily. A strong infusion can be used externally as a lotion.

EVERYDAY ILLNESSES THAT RESPOND WELL TO HERBAL MEDICINE

Y ou will have the best chances of success with herbal remedies if you can use them in the context of the following two principles of natural healing:

1. Allow rest for both the body and mind – this will create the best medium for the natural healing powers of the body to perform their work.
2. Take only a light "cleansing" diet – the process of digestion is very hard work for the body, requiring the diversion of a large part of the blood flow to the digestive organs. Let the body's priority be to carry this blood to the organs affected by the illness. Take plenty of fluids, and eat mainly fruit and vegetables for a day or two. Avoid fats and proteins, except where there has been a lot of tissue damage: proteins will be needed to form the replacement tissue. This must of course be adapted to the needs of the individual. If fruit and vegetables are found to be too indigestible reduce their intake and replace with light soups, and small amounts of cereal foods.

NOTE: **Some illnesses are so complex and variable that they may require professional treatment – in this chapter these are marked with an asterisk★**

ACNE

Acne (over-activity of the oil-producing glands of the skin) is often connected with a hormone disturbance which may need professional treatment. Before taking this step, ensure that your diet is plain and simple, with plenty of cleansing fruits and vegetables. The alterative and eliminating remedies are the most useful: try **Burdock, Nettles, Yellow Dock root and Echinacea.** These will help to clear irritating waste products from the skin; **Echinacea** has a useful anti-infective action to combat the

Acne: burdock, nettles, yellow dock and echinacea

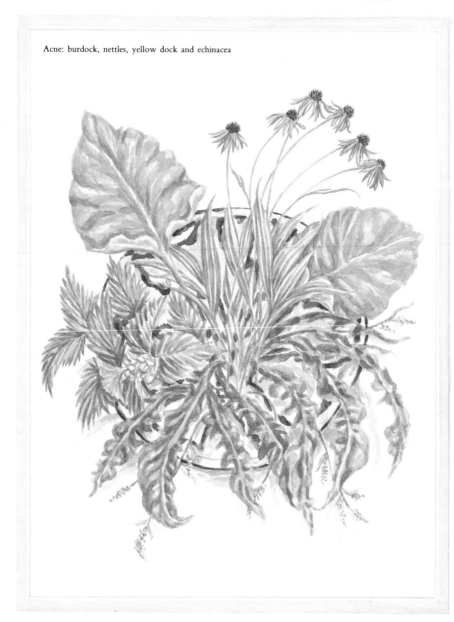

bacteria which feed on the skin secretions. **Witch Hazel**, applied to the skin, will help to reduce excess oiliness.

*ALLERGY

A wide-ranging subject, as the allergenic substances can form an endless list: food, clothing, chemical pollution or natural airborne substances can all trigger an inappropriate reaction by the body's immune system, as if something harmful was attacking the body. The symptoms are also very varied, such as the frequent asthma/eczema syndrome or hay fever, digestive disturbances, some types of arthritis, and even nervous and emotional problems. Unless it is a very obvious, clear-cut reaction, a lot of detective work may be required.

Some relief may be obtained by improving the function of the digestive system. This helps to promote the complete breakdown of any food substances which might cause an allergic reaction if absorbed while only partly digested. **Meadowsweet** and **Dandelion root** should help here, plus a bitter tonic such as **Hops**. Also, **Chamomile** is a soothing, anti-inflammatory herb to calm any reaction, either internally or locally.

*ARTHRITIS

The cause is still unknown in many cases, but the herbalist's approach is to cleanse the body of any potentially irritating toxins with herbs like **Celery seed** and **Devil's Claw**. Antacid and anti-inflammatory herbs like **Meadowsweet** and **White Willow bark** will help in a lot of cases, and in addition, **Feverfew leaves**, taken for at least 3 months to get the maximum benefit, are well worth trying. **Bladderwrack** can be used to make a soothing poultice.

A plain whole-food diet is *very* important: acidic foods must be avoided – these include sharp-tasting foods and refined carbohydrates, which have acidic end-products. A high fluid level is necessary to "flush out" the irritants.

BILIOUS ATTACK

This is a traditional name for acute disturbances of the stomach and liver, the symptoms being discomfort and nausea progressing to vomiting. There may be an associated headache, possibly migraine (see also under **MIGRAINE**). The most useful remedies

Arthritis: white willow bark, meadowsweet and celery seed

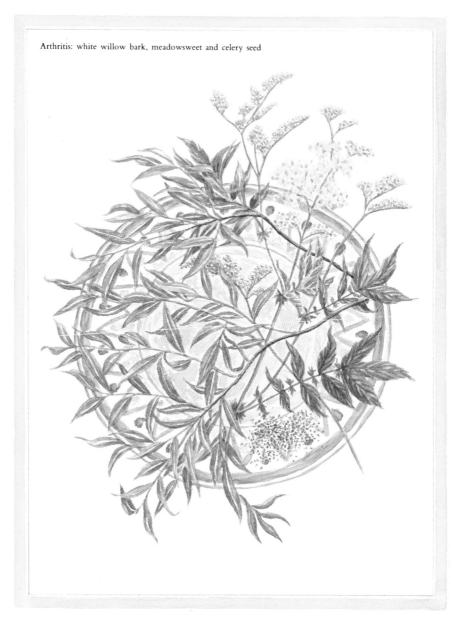

are those that soothe the stomach, such as **Slipper Elm** and **Marshmallow. Meadowseet** is a general remedy for stomach disturbances, and the liver will be specifically helped by **Dandelion root**. If it is thought that an infection is the cause, then **Garlic** and **Golden Seal** will help overcome it.

An adequate fluid intake is more important than solid food, particularly if vomiting is pronounced.

BOILS

These are infections developing at the base of the hair shaft, usually due to extremely virulent bacteria. The herbalist's approach is to clear the infection and also to aid the series of processes that the body goes through to fight off the infection, then to return the infected tissue to a normal, healthy state of functioning. Remedies that will help destroy the bacteria when applied locally are **Myrrh** and **Garlic** and, when taken internally, they stimulate the body's own immune response.

Cleansing remedies that help support the body's removal of the waste products of the inflammation include **Burdock, Cleavers** and **Echinacea** (which is another antiseptic in itself).

A poultice made of **Slippery Elm powder** and **Chickweed** will help draw the infection to the surface of the skin, allowing for an easier discharge of pus – this is a necessary, if unpleasant, aspect of the cleansing process.

BRUISING

If the skin seems to bruise too easily, the blood vessels may be very fragile. They can be strengthened with Vitamin C and rutin, a bioflavinoid, both of which are necessary in the formation of the fibers that give strength to the walls of the blood vessels. If the bruises are normal, for example if the sufferer takes part in a lot of active sports, the bruising and swelling can be reduced to a minimum by applying **Witch Hazel** to the injured area as soon as possible. This should be followed up with an application of **Arnica** which helps disperse the products of the blood leakage, which then return to the circulation.

BURNS

Only minor burns should be treated without medical attention. The first treatment should always be immersion in cold water to take the heat out of the skin and reduce the swelling. Secondly, apply an astringent like **Witch Hazel** to form a fine protective coating over the damaged skin. Thirdly, when the discomfort has been eased by this action, a healing remedy, such as **Marigold** or **St. John's Wort**, makes a good application. If an infection develops, seek professional help.

CATARRH

A common problem in places where the air is damp and/or polluted. There may be an infection present, or this may have cleared to leave the sensitive mucous membranes in a state of long-term irritation and excess mucous production. This may affect the nasal membranes, the sinus passages, the throat or lungs (where it may be diagnosed as chronic bronchitis). The first step is to treat any infection – with **Myrrh** or **Garlic**. The circulation must be considered, as this nourishes and cleanses the affected tissues – stimulants such as **Ginger, Chillies** or the more moderate **Angelica** can be used to counteract a tendency to coldness and sluggish circulation. Cleansing the body of accumulated toxins will be helped by **Echinacea** and **Cleavers**, plus liver remedies such as **Dandelion root. Elderflowers, Cudweed** and **Golden Rod** will also help in most cases.

Catarrh, or phlegm, in the lungs can be cleared with the use of expectorant remedies – see entry for **COUGHS**.

★CHEST INFECTIONS

Anti-infective remedies like **Myrrh, Garlic, Thyme** and **Balm of Gilead** will help when taken by mouth: alternatively **Thyme, Balm of Gilead** and **Aniseed** can be used as a steam inhalation. Any infected phlegm should be expelled from the lungs with expectorant remedies – see entry for **COUGHS**. If the appetite is badly affected and there is general debility, **Vervain** is an excellent convalescent restorative.

CHILBLAINS AND POOR CIRCULATION

When the hands and feet become cold due to a low external temperature, the small blood vessels constrict to conserve warmth within the center of the body. This is particularly pronounced in people who have a poor circulation to start with, and may result in the tender, swollen reddish patches of skin called chilblains. They can be avoided with the use of circulatory stimulants such as **Chillies, Ginger** and the milder **Angelica** taken internally. The first two can also be made into infusions, and added to hand and footbaths, to "draw" the blood supply down to the extremities. This needs to be done regularly to gain maximum benefit, and will also bring relief from the type of night cramps that are due to poor circulation.

The second group of useful remedies are those that open up the circulation to the skin, such as **Yarrow, Elderflowers** and **Limeflowers**.

COLDS

There is no way to avoid the sequence of symptoms associated with a head cold once the virus takes hold, but herbal medicine provides one of the most effective approaches to speeding up and resolving the whole illness. The principle, as usual, is to help the body's attempts to overcome the infection naturally, and resting, to avoid "distracting" it with any other demanding work. The immune system can be supported with **Garlic** and **Echinacea**, while the circulatory system, which may initially generate a fever to create a hostile environment for the virus, can be helped with **Ginger** or **Composition Essence**. To help break the fever, and to stimulate sweating as a cleansing mechanism for the skin, **Elderflower, Peppermint, Hyssop** or **Yarrow** can be used. A very light diet, or preferably a fruit-only diet for one or two days, is extremely helpful at the first sign of symptoms developing.

★COLIC

This very painful abdominal condition is due to spasm of the muscles of the intestines. It usually results from irritation of the sensitive mucous lining by hard particles of food, excessively strong laxatives, or certain micro-organisms in cases of infection. It is literally a "cramp" in the intestines, and is soothed by those sweet aromatic remedies whose volatile oils ease both irritation in the mucous membranes and help to relax the painful "knots" in the muscles. **Chamomile, Cinnamon, Caraway, Cardamon** and **Fennel** all make very pleasant and effective drinks, and are mild enough, in weak infusion, to give to very young children. If lactating mothers take a fairly strong infusion of the last three herbs mentioned above, it will help to stimulate milk supply and some traces of the oils will be passed on to the baby via the breast milk helping the baby's digestion naturally.

CONSTIPATION

The first line of treatment for this complaint should be dietary: a diet with plenty of whole grains and fresh fruit and vegetables is essential. Also, the stimulus of regular exercise is a great help. The normal activity of the bowel depends on alternating contraction and relaxation of its muscles: if the balance is lost in either of these phases, constipation will result. A sluggish, underactive bowel can be toned and stimulated with **Cascara**, or for a stronger action, **Senna** (recommended for temporary use only). These are best combined with the anti-colic remedies, as they may cause excessive irritation to a sensitive digestive system. If the constipation is due to too much tension and spasm in the muscles, then relaxing remedies are required: **Chamomile** and **Lemon Balm** will help, but a severe case may need professional treatment.

COUGHS

When the airways in the lungs become irritated – usually by an infection, allergy, or pollution – coughing is the normal response. It is the lungs' attempt to expel the cause of the problem.

A protective mucus is produced by the lining of the lungs to engulf any irritants. This is then transported up through the main airways, and is finally coughed up as phlegm.

This has a great cleansing benefit, as mucus remaining stagnant in the lungs is a sitting target for further infection, and of course may restrict the efficiency of breathing by covering up the oxygen-absorbing surfaces in the lungs. So, although coughing up phlegm is an unpleasant symptom, it is most important as a step towards resolving disease of the lungs.

In some chest problems characterized by a dry cough, the phlegm cannot be expelled, and expectorant remedies such as **Coltsfoot, White Horehound** and **Elecampane root** will be very useful for soothing and loosening a "tight" chest.

If the problem causing the cough is in the throat, or the voice is hoarse, a steam inhalation with **Friar's Balsam, Chamomile** or **Thyme** will be very soothing.

DANDRUFF

This is a type of eczema associated with the glands producing the natural lubricating fluid of the scalp, known as sebum. It may vary from a mild flaking of tiny patches of skin, to severe inflammation and discomfort. Internal remedies are as for **eczema**, plus a local application of **Nettle** and **Rosemary** as a strong infusion may help. This can be used daily, or may be added to hair-rinsing water in mild cases.

DEBILITY

This term implies a general "below par" feeling – tiredness and weakness as in convalescent states – many people feel this way without any association with a specific illness. Convalescent tonics include **Vervain** and **Betony**. As well as medicine, rest is important as the body's natural ally during the recovery period.

If there is no specific illness, diet and life-style must be considered. The healthy body needs the right food – plenty of fresh fruit and vegetables, moderate amounts of whole-grain cereals, whether meat or dairy products. This regime will not over burden the digestive and eliminative organs. Exercise is a vital stimulus to the body – to keep the circulation, digestion and eliminative organs in good condition, and to help counteract stress and obesity. Remedies which may help restore strength and vitality include **Betony** and **Damiana**, and the simple food **Oats** – taken as porridge, muesli, oatcakes or flapjacks.

*DEPRESSION

This is rarely a simple matter of "feeling down" – the cause may be rooted in a physical, or more commonly psychological, problem that may require great professional skill and some time to identify and correct. Herbal treatment during this period can help support the nervous system to withstand any emotional or psychological difficulties the patient may be confronting. The remedies for **DEBILITY** are suitable, plus any others specific to problem areas, such as the digestion (very commonly affected by nervous problems) or liver if orthodox drug treatment has been tried. A good diet is invaluable in this case as the nervous system has high nutritional requirements. Physical exercise (which may not be welcome) is highly recommended, to keep body functions normal, rather than allowing a slide into inactivity and debility.

DIARRHEA

The principal aim must be to find the cause of the diarrhea, which is an attempt by the digestive system to rid itself of its contents. It is a natural protective mechanism in cases of infection, or irritation from unsuitable foods, when the harmful substance is "better out than in". The disadvantage of over-activity of the bowel is that the body may lose a dangerously large amount of fluid and minerals. It can also be very uncomfortable and irritating to the lining of the digestive tract to have food passing through too rapidly.

Severe cases can be eased with astringent herbs – **Avens** has a very reliable effect, plus **Agrimony** to a milder degree. **Slippery Elm powder** will help because of its soothing mucilaginous properties, as will **Marshmallow root. Meadowsweet** flowers are specific for diarrhea in children, and the leaves will help as a general aid to the digestive system in adults.

★DYSPEPSIA

This term covers a wide range of disturbances of the stomach, from mild uncomfortable flatulence, through the burning pains of over-acidity and indigestion, to the more worrying problem of a suspected ulcer. If the problem is either severe or long-lasting, professional treatment must be sought. In milder cases, however, keep to a plain, light diet, and take the following herbal remedies, which should bring relief to most sufferers: **Slippery Elm** and **Marshmallow root** will soothe the lining of an irritated stomach; **Meadowsweet, Lemon Balm** and **Chamomile** have other anti-inflammatory benefits; **Hops** and **Vervain** will help stimulate a sluggish digestion, if this is responsible for the problem. **Fennel, Ginger** and **Caraway** are most useful for flatulence.

*ECZEMA

Eczema is a complex problem, and requires much detective work into the possible causes. As a result, there are few remedies which apply to every case. The best general approach is to use initially the "cleansing" remedies, with the intention of eliminating any toxins which may be irritating a sensitive skin. **Dandelion root, Cleavers, Nettles** and **Oregon Grape** help through stimulating the liver, kidneys and lymphatic system (part of the circulation). Other causes may be found in the nervous system, digestive and immune systems, and must be treated accordingly: stress and food allergies are frequently involved.

See **SKIN IRRITATION** for remedies which apply to the skin.

EYE IRRITATION

Bloodshot, watery, itchy eyes can be due to several causes, such as infections, allergies and exposure to airborne irritants (smoke or chemical fumes). **Eyebright** is an astringent remedy which has been used for hundreds of years. It has a toning effect on the surface of the eye, and may be combined with **Golden Seal** to make an anti-infective eyewash.

HEMORRHOIDS

These varicose veins around the anus may be the result of increased internal abdominal pressure, often a result of constipation or pregnancy, or due to excess tension in the ring of muscle at the opening of the anus that closes off the bowel between evacuations. Constipation must be avoided, as the first line of treatment, then local applications of astringent remedies, notably **Witch Hazel** and **Lesser Celandine**, will be very soothing.

*HEADACHES

Unless these are obviously due to problems such as stress or tiredness, professional attention should be sought to rule out any more serious causes.

Rest and relaxation generally help, and relaxing remedies such as **Chamomile, Passiflora, Valerian** and particularly **Betony** will aid recovery. Nerve tonics such as **Damiana** and **Vervain** may be useful in the treatment of long-term stress.

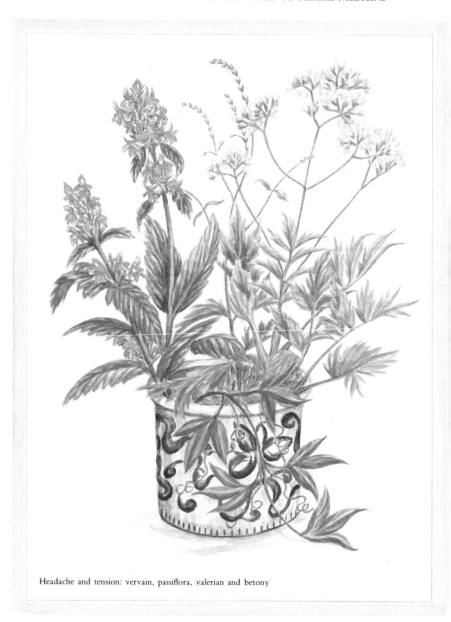

Headache and tension: vervain, passiflora, valerian and betony

*HEART PROBLEMS

Do not seek to treat heart problems without professional attention. there are several remedies which make a useful addition to professional treatment and which are compatible with orthodox drugs. **Hawthorn** and **Motherwort** have a tonic, almost nourishing, influence on the heart and blood vessels – they will strengthen the heart without influencing its rate. If the heart is struggling against high blood pressure, **Yarrow** and **Limeflowers** will help to normalize the blood pressure *and* strengthen the walls of the blood vessels. **Garlic** helps to mobilize fatty deposits from the bloodstream *and* will reduce the clotting tendency which may occur within damaged linings of blood vessels.

INFLUENZA

Treat as for **COLDS** and **CHEST INFECTIONS.** Bear in mind that the convalescent stage, when rest is indicated, is most important: **debility** and **depression** can be severe at this time.

MENSTRUAL PROBLEMS

Heavy or painful periods can be eased by **Black Haw, Motherwort** and **Raspberry leaves** – these have a tonic and relaxing influence on the muscle of the womb. In addition, **Chamomile** and **Passiflora** may help to reduce pain. If the disturbances are due to the onset of the menopause, then **St. John's Wort** is a useful addition.

MIGRAINE

This unpleasant headache can be associated with disturbances of vision and/or digestive upsets. It can be caused by different foods, stress and tension, or missing a meal – so the remedies used in the treatment can vary widely. The single most helpful remedy is **Feverfew**, which seems to alleviate the tightening of the blood vessels in the brain which causes the basic disturbance. This is a preventative rather than curative treatment, so it will take at least 2 or 3 months to achieve maximum benefit. It should be taken every day during this time.

To ease the pain once it has started, relaxing remedies such as **Passiflora, Chamomile** and **Lemon Balm** are recommended – the last two will also help to settle any stomach problems.

NERVOUS TENSION

There are few people who are able to avoid stress in modern society. The body's natural response to stress is a "fight or flight" reaction – hardly suitable for the sort of problems most common today. We will feel less taut after using up the energy that the "fight or flight" reaction prepares us for – swimming, cycling, even walking, helps the body to relax and eases tension.

If exercise is not sufficient to counteract the stress, anxiety, tension, or insomnia, the herbal relaxants such as **Passiflora, Valerian** and **Lavender** will help. If the problem has got to the stage of nervous exhaustion, the restoratives **Vervain, Betony** and **Damiana**, are recommended.

SINUSITIS

Congestion of the mucous membrane-lined cavities of the skull can be a persistent and very unpleasant problem, causing head-aches, catarrhal deafness and dizziness. Infections here can be very difficult to clear: **Garlic** and **Echinacea** give the best results. The circulation must be efficient, so use **Ginger** or **Angelica** if it is at all sluggish. Eliminatory functions must also work well; try **Dandelion root** to ensure good liver function.

A useful lotion to apply over the affected sinuses is made from a combination of **Myrrh, Cayenne** and **Golden Seal**. Avoid getting it in the eyes – it is very irritating to sensitive membranes.

SKIN IRRITATION

Irritation of the skin is caused by a number of factors. The best internal treatment is a cleansing regime, as recommended for **ECZEMA**. Locally, the most soothing applications for itchy or inflamed skin are **Marigold, Chickweed** or **St. John's Wort** – all available as creams or ointments. I have also found pure Vitamin E oil to be very useful for dry, inflamed skins.

SUNBURN

The first line of treatment for sunburn is to soak the affected area with **Distilled Witch Hazel**. Place a square of lint, or similar sterile, absorbent fabric, over the area, and pour on the witch hazel; continue adding witch hazel to prevent the lint from drying out. This forms a protective layer over the damaged skin which prevents the entry of infections and reduces the pain and inflammation. Follow up by applying wheatgerm oil, or pure Vitamin E oil – this helps to moisturize the skin and reduces the amount of damage, thus facilitating the healing process.

THROAT INFECTIONS

Gargles and mouthwashes will soothe the affected area and help reduce the infection. **Myrrh, Red Sage, Thyme** and **Golden Seal** are the most useful remedies. **Garlic** and **Echinacea** can be taken internally to promote the immune system's reaction to the infection. If the condition is very painful, **Raspberry leaves** and **Eyebright** infusions, sipped, will reduce the discomfort. **Marshmallow root**, when sipped, also has a soothing effect.

THRUSH

Thrust is related to both yeasts and fungi and is present on the body surface at all times. Symptoms first appear when it overcomes the body's defences, which normally check its spread. Mucous membranes in the mouth (particularly in young children), the vagina and the digestive system can all be affected. Treat by cutting out the refined sugar in your diet – this helps to starve the sugar-loving thrush organism. Eat live natural yogurt, as the acids create a hostile environment for thrush, and apply it to the vagina if necessary. Use anti-infective remedies, such as **Marigold, Myrrh** and **Echinacea**, as a mouthwash or douche. These can also be sipped for internal benefit. The irritation can be relieved by astringents such as **Raspberry leaves** for the mouth, or **Witch Hazel** for the vagina.

TRAVEL SICKNESS

This unpleasant feeling of nausea, sometimes with actual vomiting and faintness, is due to the disorientation of the sense of balance during travelling. It can be settled by taking small regular doses of **Ginger** before and during the journey. Other remedies include **Passiflora**, which helps to reduce the disturbance to the nervous system (take this on the previous day, as well as the day of traveling), plus **Meadowsweet** for its direct benefit on the stomach.

*URINARY PROBLEMS

Only the most straightforward of urinary disorders should be treated without professional attention – the cleansing action of the kidneys is essential to good health and life itself. However, relatively minor (though very unpleasant) problems, such as recurrent cystitis, or persistent discomfort and the need to pass water frequently, respond well to herbal treatment. If there is a chance that an infection is causing problems, diuretic remedies to "flush through" the urinary system, such as **Dandelion leaf** and **Horsetail**, will help. Ensure that there is a good fluid intake to make this easier – including lemon juice diluted with hot water and honey to sweeten, if required. **Echinacea** and **Golden Seal** will strengthen the body's general resistance to infection. The specific anti-infective remedies for the urinary system are **Celery seed** and **Bearberry**.

If the irritation is not due to an infection, **Dandelion leaves, Horsetail** and **Celery seed** are still useful as cleansing and soothing remedies for the urinary tract. If a chill has brought on the problem, try **Ginger** or **Angelica**, or, in the case of nervous tension irritating the bladder, **Passiflora** or **Valerian** should help.

VARICOSE VEINS

These over-stretched blood vessels have lost their ability to return blood efficiently from the tissues of the body to the main veins – the "trunk roads" that return blood to the heart. The legs are the worst affected area because here the veins are constantly working against the force of gravity, which tends to push the blood back towards the feet. People who are standing still most of the day are most susceptible. Other causes of increased abdominal pressure, such as constipation and pregnancy, may further add to the problem. Sufferers should try to counteract these influences by sitting with the feet raised when possible, and making the calf muscles work by flexing and stretching the ankle, thus causing a pumping action in the lower leg.

Weakness in the blood vessels may be improved with **Hawthorn, Yarrow** and **Golden Seal**. Excess fluid at the ankle can be helped with gentle massage – and with **Dandelion leaf** to

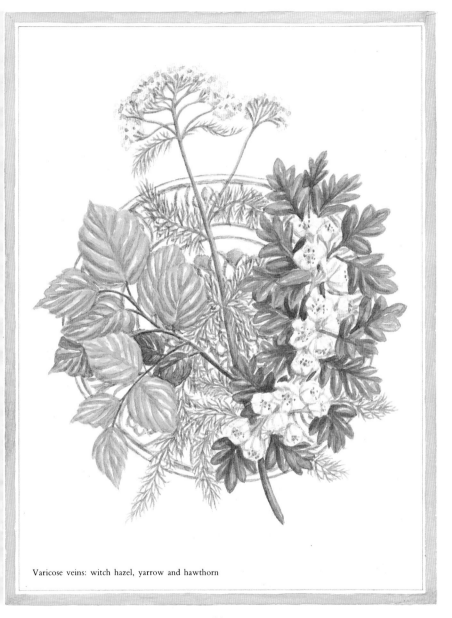

Varicose veins: witch hazel, yarrow and hawthorn

stimulate kidney function. A healing, astringent lotion made from **Witch Hazel** and **Marigold** can be applied to the veins to ease discomfort.

WARTS

These outgrowths of skin may be caused by a virus. They can appear and disappear with no apparent explanation – sometimes charms and folk remedies work as well as any medicine! The most reliable herbal treatment is the application of the fresh juice of the **Greater Celandine**. If this plant is unavailable, the juice of the **Dandelion** is the next best thing.

★WOUNDS

The first requirement with any wound is to staunch the blood flow – this can be done by placing a sterile pad of lint over the wound and holding it firmly in place for a few minutes. Herbal remedies which help with their astringent action are **Yarrow** and **Witch Hazel**.

The wound should be inspected to ensure that it is clear: flushing it over with dilute **Tincture of Myrrh** will prevent any infections from developing. When a hard scab or crust has formed, and any inflammation is starting to abate, **Marigold, St. John's Wort** and **Comfrey** will help promote the healing process. **Comfrey** is also reputed to help minimize the formation of scar tissue.

FURTHER READING

A good traditional herbal, wider in scope than this book as it includes more herbs, plus points on, for example, cosmetic preparations, and folklore, is *A Modern Herbal* by Mrs. M. Grieve – it is available in paperback, published by Penguin.

For readers interested more specifically in medical herbalism, *The Dictionary of Modern Herbalism* by Simon Mills FNIMH, published by Thorsons, is excellent. For those thinking of a career in herbal medicine, *Herbal Medicine* by Fritz Weiss, published by Beaconsfield Arcanum, is a good introduction to the professional viewpoint.

The School of Herbal Medicine and Phytotherapy, at 148 Forest Road, Tunbridge Wells, Kent, runs a one-year correspondence course for laypeople with an interest in herbal medicine, and also courses of longer duration which train students to professional standards.

Further information about the National Institute of Medical Herbalists can be obtained from the Secretary, National Institute of Medical Herbalists, 41 Hatherley Road, Winchester, Hampshire SO22 6RR.

INDEX

Page numbers in italics refer to illustrations